UNDERSTANDING DIABETES FOR ACTION

UNDERSTANDING DIABETES FOR ACTION

RETHINKING HOW YOU HANDLE DIABETES
A HOLISTIC APPROACH

… no such thing as insulin resistance

Roland Fleurizier, ND

SUBMITTED TO TRINITY SCHOOL OF NATURAL HEALTH, 220 PARKER STREET, WARSAW, IN 46580, USA,

IN PARTIAL FULFILLMENT OF THE REQUIREMENTS FOR THE DOCTOR OF NATUROPATHY DEGREE

authorHOUSE®

AuthorHouse™
1663 Liberty Drive
Bloomington, IN 47403
www.authorhouse.com
Phone: 833-262-8899

Published by AuthorHouse   03/09/2021

ISBN: 978-1-4918-4224-9 (sc)
ISBN: 978-1-4918-4225-6 (e)

Library of Congress Control Number: 2013922685

Print information available on the last page.

ACKNOWLEDGEMENTS

This work would not have been possible without the unconditional support of many people. I must begin by thanking Professor Susan Schoettmer for her immediate approval of the dissertation prospectus, which was the boost to start this study.

I must also thank Joseph Desrosiers, N.D., Jean Anthony Archer, N.D, Geuns Eustache, N.D., M.H., Rochenel Charles ND, MH and other health practitioners in the New York City area, such as Enold Millen, ND, Marie André Ménard, CNHP, who truthfully answered all my questions throughout the interviews.

Special appreciation is due to Ding Wei-Cheng as he dedicated himself to assess the adaptation and coherence of the statistical procedures presented in this study.

I express many thanks to Professor David Levin who has not bargained his editing knowledge, without which the dissertation could not have been completed in the scheduled time.

J'exprime ma gratitude à mon épouse, Marie Denise Fleurizier, pour sa disponibilité permanente, à ma fille Rivkie E. Fleurizier et à mon fils Gary N. Fleurizier, tous deux source intarissable d'affection et d'optimisme et témoins infatigables, comme leur mère, de mes nuits de veille.

Special thanks go also to all those who one way or another, worked thoughtfully or intuitively towards the achievement of this dissertation.

Roland Fleurizier, ND

This study would not have been completed without the help and support of all the aforementioned. I am therefore presenting to them my genuine gratitude.

I also owe a debt of gratitude to those participants in my health class and to clients whose thoughtful questions and personal health needs inspired and encouraged the writing of UNDERSTANDING DIABETES FOR ACTION.

CONTENTS

Chapter 2

Chapter 3

Chapter 4

CHAPTER 1

BACKGROUND OF THE STUDY

My mid-1980s Haitian internship with the late Dr. Lamarque Douyon, a well-known psychiatrist in the country's capital city of Port-au-Prince, Haiti, sparked my penchant for psychosomatic medicine. This health practitioner was one of the professors who naturally encouraged my inclination for clinical psychology during my last year of psychology studies at the Faculty of Ethnology.

Later on, in New York, Dr. Joseph Desrosiers, a distinguished Naturopathic Kinesiologist in the Haitian community, observed that I had a scar in the brain, which I was unaware of as I never had any headache, not realizing that people could have scar tissues, misalignments, blood leaks, dried blood, dead blood, etc. in the brain without any symptoms. Afterwards, I had similar experiences, especially since three siblings were involved in a car accident. By means of Applied or Clinical Kinesiology, dried blood was found on the brain of one of them, but a CAT-scan had not discovered it.

I found about Applied Kinesiology (AK) through Dr. Desrosiers, as this profession can only be learned thoroughly after months or even years of practice. Applied or Clinical Kinesiology is the science of testing the muscles to "search for the underlying causes of the apparent symptoms."[1] It allows the health kinesiology practitioner to uncover the exact cause of a symptom or imbalance, whether it be physical, emotional, or spiritual. In fact, some muscles

---

[1] Your Body Can Talk—The Art and Application of Clinical Kinesiology—by Susan L. Levy, D. C. and Carl Lehr, M.A.—1996

may be temporarily out of balance due to a deficiency of certain vitamins, minerals, or trace elements. As a complementary approach to naturopathy, kinesiology can often help to restore health balance.

My dedication and passion for natural and energy medicine is an extension of various experiences accumulated to date, mostly in homeopathic medicine and Applied Kinesiology, after I had previously received three undergraduate degrees, two masters, and earned an admission to a doctoral program.

Much has been said about diabetes. The way to tackle it is even largely unknown to most physicians. It seems that diabetics do not fully comprehend all of the aspects of their ailment. For the most part diabetes has been considered to be a lifetime condition. With this in mind, I have decided to undertake this research to initiate a comprehensive, restorative agenda for diabetics to use in order to subjugate their disease and prevent the complications outlined in the recommendations.

This research work is a continuation of the Gretchen Scalpi[2] reported theory regarding pre-diabetes and diabetes. Her theory states that pre-diabetics have a blood sugar level ranging anywhere from 100 and 125 mg/dl, and that diabetics have a blood sugar level above 125 mg/dl or "a causal blood sugar level, usually after eating, greater than or equal to 200 mg/dl."

This study draws on the work of the late Dr. Christopher D. Saudek,[3] former president of the American Diabetes Association and Director of the Johns Hopkins Diabetes Center. He agreed that Type-I diabetes is due to the complete destruction of pancreatic beta cells by means of immune mechanisms.

In drawing also on the work of Jennie Brand-Miller, Kaye Foster-Powell, Alan W. Barclay, and Stephen Colagiuri, who all recommend plenty of vegetables, legumes, rice, pasta, noodles, and

---

[2]   She published in 2011 "The Everything Guide to Managing and Reversing Pre-Diabetes."

[3]   In 1997, he coauthored "The Johns Hopkins Guide to Diabetes: for Today and Tomorrow."

fruits in the diet of youngsters with Type-I Diabetes, this study aims to generate a new protocol for the reversal of diabetes.

Some people were born with the diabetes ailment; others acquired it from some very complex processes that are further described in this study. Factors that may be involved in the diabetes acquisition are multitudinous. Some health practitioners, including physicians, hold misleading views on how to best deal with diabetes. This study therefore takes into account the profusion of views by scholars on diabetes.

Statement of the Problem

In a society where vitality and creativity ought to prevail, access to the fast food industry is unremitted, and most adults and children alike have developed a fascination for the convenience of unbalanced meals. Yet the consumption of unhealthy foods can easily shut down the entire body, predominantly the functions of the brain. As a result, the blood glucose may rise beyond the normal range, which is 98-100, and even go over 125, apparently leaving insulin as the sole "remedy." Yet insulin intake actually increases the chance of being obese since it causes fat build-up around the body's middle line. Therefore, lacking exercise and adequate nutrition to lessen fat build-up, many children today are diagnosed with adult Type 2 diabetes. This generation of children may not outlive their parents.

The Significance of the Study

Proper nutrition could be vital to nearly everyone with diabetes. Existing studies inadequately address this issue and there are conflicting conclusions which keep the debate alive. Consequently, this study attempts to provide guidance for a new approach to manage and even reverse diabetes. Information brought forth in this study might be grounds for implementing changes in the area of natural health and more precisely for creating a new health protocol for diabetic patients. Once this is done, health recovery and contentment should increase.

Research Questions

This study mainly examines correlations between food ingestion, heredity, the hepatic system, the glandular system, vitamin and/or mineral deficiencies and diabetes by responding to the following questions:

1. Is diabetes a direct function of food consumption?
2. Is diabetes a direct result of heredity?
3. Is diabetes a direct result of malfunction of the hepatic system?
4. Is diabetes a direct result of malfunction of the glandular system?
5. Is diabetes a direct result of vitamin and/or mineral deficiencies?
6. Can contingent factors (such as free radicals, stress, dehydration, and emotions) lead to hyperglycemia?

A contingent factor is something that can either directly cause the disease or contribute to it. Dehydration, stress, and emotions, for instance, can each be either a contributor to disease or the originator of the disease.

Limitations of the Study

Family history, age, race or ethnicities have no specific bearing on the development of the diabetes ailment. They are considered extraneous variables and are not part of this study. The rationale for this is that siblings subjected to similar diets and sedentary lifestyles are likely to develop the same diseases if genetic predispositions are present.

Definition of Operational Terms

The research questions imply a causal relationship among these variables: food consumption, obesity, and diabetes. A variable is defined as a varying concept. Heredity, hepatic system malfunction, and glandular system malfunction, or vitamin and mineral deficiencies either together or separately may have an impact on the dependent variable: diabetes. Therefore, the research questions are restated using at a minimum, a multi independent variable relationship to diabetes, the only dependent variable in this study.

What Is Diabetes?

Diabetes is an ailment alternatively labeled gestational, Type-I, or Type-II—depending on the degree of starvation of the human body for the hormone insulin to normalize the excessive rise of carbohydrates in the blood. However, gestational diabetes, Type-I and Type-II diabetes are not variables in this study. Each one of them simply describes a possible category (an attribute) of the variable diabetes, even though each of the major types of diabetes may deal with the intensity or amount of insulin ingestion.

What is Heredity?

Heredity is the transmission of genetic materials from ancestors to their descendants.

Ancestors may be defined as great-grandparents and beyond. Descendants are children, grandchildren, or great-grandchildren of the ancestors. A hereditary disease such as diabetes may be acquired if any parents, grandparents, or great-grand parents had developed it during their lifetime, which would predispose any descendants to acquire such ailment due to a genetic weakness. In other words, descendants may have been deficient at birth; that is, their body may not have been absorbing chromium, which in the most severe cases, may create a need for constant inoculation of insulin.

Mineral and Vitamin Deficiencies

Minerals and vitamins assure a daily nutritional ingestion for proper body function. Just like proteins, they are said to be the "building blocks" of the body. A deficiency in vitamins and/or minerals can perturb bodily biochemical activities, and eventually alter blood sugar.

Glandular System

The glandular system is the body system that is responsible for hormone secretions, which sends signals to body parts to ensure proper functions. Endocrine glands release their secretions directly into the bloodstream, which largely impact body metabolism.[4]

Hepatic System

The hepatic system is composed of the liver, one of the main organs of the digestive system due to its metabolic functions. A dysfunction of the liver may undermine the wholeness of the body as much as any systemic disease.

Stress and Emotions

Stress is a state of mind that affects the nerves and causes the stressed person to burn much more vitamin B12 than usual. Stress makes the body acidic; fear or emotions can be a direct result of stress, causing the heart to beat faster and deliver more blood and oxygen to the muscles. The intensity of fear or emotions behind the stress can create a desire for more body fuels, such as sugar and fat. Henceforth stress is an originator of diseases.

Dehydration

Lack of drinking water or any intestinal bacteria or virus that may undermine either fluid distribution or water assimilation are part of the possible causes of dehydration. Dehydration can disrupt biochemical activities and trigger blood sugar variations.

Summary: The theories that inspired and accompanied this text are cited as a framework in the beginning of this chapter. Further, the concepts that go into the groundwork of this study are precisely defined to avoid confusions and misinterpretations.

---

[4]   Metabolism is a life—preserving biochemical activity during which ingested food is converted into energy and other needed products or substances.

CHAPTER 2

LITERATURE REVIEW

Most of the literature relevant to natural health dates back from the early 1950s through the present. The debate concerning natural health has gone through various discourses on enzymes, diet and nutrition, vitamins and minerals, amino acids, food supplements, and medications, which are likely to affect in one way or another the overall health of humans. Therefore the literature review involves hundreds of books and articles in scholarly journals. Since the literature review focuses on the most pertinent work that already exists, this study points out areas for improving and even correcting diabetes.

What Does it Mean to be Overweight or Obese?

Until recently, it was assumed that obesity is a causative factor and perhaps even the only causative factor of diabetes. It had also been assumed that this ailment was preventable, but irreversible. However, it is becoming evident that diabetes is more frequent in those who have excess weight or are obese. Obesity can damage the hormones that control blood sugar and therefore harmfully influence almost every cell and organ in a person's body, particularly the heart and lungs, muscles and bones, kidneys and digestive tract, etc. But what does it mean to be overweight or obese?

Being overweight or obese is to retain excessive fat. This can be estimated through the calculation of the body mass index (BMI), which is an estimation of the total body fat mass. A healthy BMI for adult individuals should be between 18.5 and 24.9.[5] However, a BMI between 25.0 and 29.9[6] is regarded as overweight and a BMI of 30 or higher is considered obese. The BMI in children and young people (adolescents) age 2 to 20 year olds is expressed in percentiles; that is, a BMI in the 85th to 94th percentiles is considered overweight for both age and gender and a BMI in the 95th percentile or higher is considered obese.[7]

Diabetes has been a recurrent problem all over the world, especially in the more developed western countries, such as the United States. The World Health Organization released statistics that show that America has a preponderance of overweight people. Joel Gittelsohn et al.[8] performed a search on diabetes and obesity status. Their findings have shown non insulin diabetes mellitus to be the leading cause of death in North America. In Canada, people who are obese and diabetic are not held responsible for consuming junk foods. Rather, stores are blamed for obesity and diabetes. Nevertheless, they found diabetes to be more prevalent among Native Americans than Canadians.

The number of adult diabetics in the United States today accounts for over 21 million,[9] which represent nearly 10% of the entire U.S. adult population. This percentage is expected to more than double by the year 2050. Many Americans are usually time constrained and hence consume many fast foods, which results in a lack of proper nutrition. It is therefore understood that, with the "convenience" of the transport system, about one third of the adult female population in the United States are obese. The Mexican, Peruvian, and Paraguayan populations are affected by obesity in the same proportions.

---

[5]   The Obesity Prevention Source: Why Use Body Mass Index? by the Harvard
      School of Public Health, 2012
[6]   The Obesity Prevention Source, op. cit.
[7]   The Obesity Prevention Source, op. cit.
[8]   The Journal of Nutrition, 1998
[9]   Volume 26, Number 1, 2008—Clinical Diabetes by Richard W. Nesto, MD

The Global Crisis of Obesity

The Organization for Economic Cooperation and Development research results[10] on obesity and economic conditions are shocking. About 70 percent of both adult American men and women are overweight or obese, and researchers predict that, all things being equal, this number will continue to increase over the next ten years. In fact, three out of every four Americans are expected to be overweight or obese by this time. This trend began during the 1980s and has steadily grown over the years, as shown on the graph that follows.

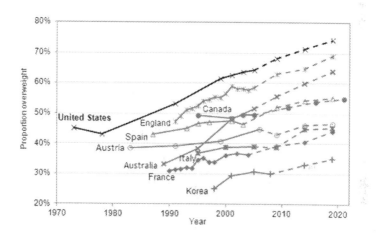

Ethnicity is insignificant in determining obesity rates, especially for women. In fact, obesity rates are higher in African-American women and in Mexican-American women compared to non-Hispanic white women by seventeen percent and six percent, respectively.[11]

40 percent of all children worldwide are overweight. This is significant, however only about half of them are obese.[12] During the last ten years, children obesity has declined, symptomatic of a

---

[10] The Journal of Nutrition, Article posted online by Marion Nestle— September 27, 2010
[11] The Journal of Nutrition, Article posted online by Marion Nestle— September 27, 2010
[12] Obesity, A New Global Epidemic: TV5Monde.org, 2006

downward trend in childhood obesity. However, Hispanic boys and African-American girls have continued to display a fifty percent higher obesity rate than white non-Hispanic boys and girls.[13]

One hundred sixty million adults in South East Asia are in danger of developing diseases that result from obesity.[14] The Middle East is no exception with respect to obesity. In fact, the obesity rates in Lebanon, Saudi Arabia, and Qatar have reached 30% of the adult population. Researchers nonetheless have observed a stabilization of obesity in Europe, with a slight decline seen in France, Denmark, Britain, Scotland, and Netherlands.

Obesity as Part of the Iceberg

In Thailand, child obesity rates have grown up from 12.2 to 15.6 percent in two years.[15] In Saudi Arabia, 17 percent of boys and 40 percent of girls are obese. In Australia, studies have shown that in 2008 Australian boys and girls are overweight or obese at the rates of 21 and 25 percent, respectively.[16] In China, 13 million children are overweight; with this figure representing 5 percent of the entire population.[17] In the United States, the rate of obesity in youngsters aged 2 to 19 has reached 17 percent.[18] All of these children may be at risk of developing Type 2 diabetes.

Childhood obesity is growing at an alarming rate worldwide, doubling every ten years. Being overweight can bring down the life expectancy of children. In Arkansas in the United States, 40 percent of children are overweight. This prompted Bill Clinton to admit that his past obsession for chips, burgers and fries of McDonald's and his appetite for pizza paved the way for his lecture "Weight of the Nation" in Washington, July 27, 2009. At that time, the country's

---

[13] Obesity, A New Global Epidemic, op. cit.
[14] Obesity, A New Global Epidemic, op. cit.
[15] World Health Organization: Global Strategy on Diet, Physical Activity and Health by DR P. PUSKA and al., 2003
[16] The Obesity Prevention Source, op. cit.
[17] Obesity, A New Global Epidemic, op. cit.
[18] No Longer Just 'Adult-Onset' published in the New York Times on May 6, 2012 based upon a new study, published in The New England Journal of Medicine

leading experts drew up an inventory of this pandemic that has been afflicting the United States for about a quarter of a century.[19]

Developing countries are hit by obesity as well. Lack of economic development and increased urban migration explain most of the explosion of obesity in those countries. Once living in towns, the villagers, economically affected, are forced to change their eating habits and have ended up eating foods low in dietetic qualities. However, overweight rates affect more women than men. Staying at home and eating excessively naturally explains much of their excess weight.

Fast-Food and Trans-Fatty Acids

The main cause of the growing phenomenon of obesity in the world was theorized in France for the first time in 1979 by husband and wife, Joel and Stella Rosnay who focused their belief on the causes of obesity by the term "junk food." They made no allusion to fast food being the major component of the overall puzzle, but still mentioned that the daily diet was too rich in fat and sugar. Joel and Stella Rosnay also pointed out that consumers who are fond of trans-fatty acids and carbohydrates are at risk of becoming hyperglycemic and developing cardiovascular diseases. Recent writing about "junk food" vehemently condemns what they call non-natural products from the processed food industry. The way to a better life is to overcome the resistance of the processed food industry.

Statistical data show the differences between the nutritional levels of vitamin C of an orange in the early 1960s and that of a contemporary orange. The British Food Journal undertook a study through laboratory research, which proposed to analyze the nutrient content of twenty-five fruits and vegetables sold in the summer of 2002 in Canadian supermarkets. For comparison, the laboratory used solely the government data for the years 1951, 1972 and 1999. The study results have shown major reductions in levels of calcium, iron, magnesium, copper and sodium in vegetables. Major

---

[19] Toxic Food by William Reymond—2007

reductions in iron, magnesium, copper, and potassium were also found in the fruits. The biggest percentage change was in the steep decline of copper in vegetables, which now account for less than 20 percent of the past amount.[20]

The Causes of the Degradation of Public Health

Public relation communications in the food industry are designed to instill doubt among consumers. They therefore repeat *ad nauseam* the same argument so as to turn it into an apparent truth, as evidence by the research results of Brian Halweil.[21] Halweil compared among other things, qualities of meat, fish and dairy products. He found that as the chickens were enriched with pork, the meat had become fatter and less rich in iron while the calcium levels of dairy products fell. A similar conclusion was evidenced for fruits (pears, oranges) and vegetables (tomatoes, carrots). According Halweil, three apples must be eaten today to get the equivalent nutrition contained in an apple from the 1960s.[22] Similarly, a 2004 study conducted by Dr. Donald Davis, a biochemist at the University of Texas, showed a reduction of vitamins and minerals in forty three selected plants.[23]

For the World Health Organization (WHO), obesity is a pandemic like AIDS, the Black Death or the Spanish flu. The author of "Toxic Food" cites McDonald's, Coca-Cola and other multinational corporations in the development of the obesity pandemic. He describes men and women of today's society as equivalent to the passengers of the Titanic as a way to emphasize the degree of peril of the health of current society.

Obesity has increased as the food industry has settled throughout all social classes, resulting in an immediate increase of

---

[20] Anne—Marie Mayer, << Historical Changes in the Mineral Content of Fruits and Vegetables>>, British Food Journal, volume 99, issue 6, http://www.californiaearthminerals.com/media/british-food-mineral-depletion-study-v101.pdf.

[21] Working under the independent association, World Watch Institute

[22] http://www.worldwatch.org

[23] The Journal of the American College of Nutrition, by Dr. Donald Davis—2004

related diseases such as Type-II diabetes.[24] Despite the obesity crisis, some elected officials believe that the current government would be out of its role if it were to challenge the American way of life by turning the obesity crisis into a political issue. This encourages the individual to eat to their heart's content and plays into the long term strategies of the food industry.

Humans living in ancient time had no choice but to take advantage of healthy eating. During the Middle Ages, for instance, rations of these people consisted of barley, oat, rye, wheat, bread, meats, vegetables, pasta, etc. Not only were most of these foods well suited to sustain human health, they were also organic and contained no additives. Therefore everything they ate could be easily digested.

Digestion and Enzymes

Most foods contain either additives or farm chemicals. As time goes by the body may build up a tolerance to additives and/or chemical materials that can damage the human body in the long run. According to the physician Hiromi Shinya, drug explanatory guides do not always mention all the side effects that the medicine is likely to generate. In fact, medications that produce instant relief are usually highly toxic and so are harmful to the body. That is why herbal medicine is designed to work gradually as the body heals itself slowly.

Drugs to treat erectile dysfunction are so toxic that they can cause swelling, nasal congestion, and breathing problems that are closed to suffocation and death. Gastrointestinal drugs or antacids, usually to treat heartburn, may lead to erectile dysfunction and male sterility due to a sudden decrease in sperm count. Heartburn and acid reflux are not disease; they each are warnings that the stomach is not secreting enough hydrochloric acid, as opposed to an over secretion of this same acid. Orthodox medicine wrongly believes, in case of heartburn, that there is hyper secretion of stomach acid, and prescribes strong antacids to restore internal balance (homeostasis). These prescriptions will shorten the lifespan of those who ingest them.

---

[24] Toxic Food by William Reymond—2007

People who are experiencing heartburn or acid reflux may have an untreated digestive condition: usually those people are not eliminating daily. As a result their body accumulates toxins, develops diverticulitis, and causes stool to stagnate and eventually rot. It stands to reason that Shinya has noticed, over the years, that most of his breast cancer patients had similar "intestinal characteristics." Thus, he concluded that a close relationship exists between breast cancer, colon cancer, and the intestinal condition.

Multiple factors cause diseases, such as lack of exercise, stress, food, water, medicine, and the living environment. The body produces new cells; depending on the body areas, and under enzyme influence, cell replacement may take several days or even years to process. Enzyme is a broad term for "a protein catalyst" that the cells of all living things manufacture, whether they are animals, plants, or humans. We need to start thinking at the cellular level, and consider that water, food, and medicine ingestion participate in cell formation to determine our health as they each affect the gastrointestinal system. We should also consider the toxicity of dead cells that are not excreted. Later on, the blood vessels, through the circulatory system, will transport all ingredients, including the nutrients and waste materials in our water, food, and drugs, to manufacture new cells—without consideration of the quality of these items.

Enzymes in excess may disturb bodily homeostasis, which creates a shortage of enzymes in other areas, and thus departs from cell repair and nervous and immune support. The body processes more than 5,000 types of enzymes. Some enzymes come from food ingestion, others, about 3,000 in number, are manufactured by intestinal bacteria when the intestinal surroundings are beneficial to enzyme production. They (enzymes) each have a specific appellation and function: gastric juice produces the enzyme pepsin, which act only in response to protein. The saliva triggers the digestive enzyme amylase to respond to starchy foods. During the digestion process enzymes are broken down for their absorption as peptides and amino acids in the intestinal tract.

Enzymes, necessary for digestion and absorption, may deplete as a result of copious consumptions of tobacco, alcohol, medicine, and food containing additives creating a shortage in some areas of the body, such as breathing, heartbeats, body movement, etc. Frequent exposure to ultraviolet rays, electromagnetic waves, and ingestion of food that liberates toxins in the colon are factors of free radical production and enzyme depletion. Another factor of enzyme depletion is chemotherapy because the body uses much of its digestive, metabolic enzymes to detoxify itself, resulting in nausea, crumbling skin, loss of hair and appetite, and a slowdown in cell metabolism.[25] No wonder that chemotherapy works against the body's natural mechanisms.

Billions of harmful bacteria enter the stomach daily through food consumption. As a defensive measure, and to destroy them, the human body maintains strong acid levels of pH 1.5 to 3.0 in the stomach and female vagina. Suppressing stomach acid with drugs allows harmful bacteria to transit untreated from the stomach to penetrate the intestines and cause various illnesses. Pepsin and hydrochloric acid secretion are suppressed whenever medications are used to suppress stomach acid secretion. This suppression of stomach acid deactivates digestive enzymes, favors indigestion, and makes it more difficult for absorption of minerals.

Stomach acid may flow up to the esophagus to create warning signs of pain and uneasiness known as heartburn or upset stomach. Factors promoting heartburn are smoking, alcohol, and coffee, overdose, and going to sleep with undigested foods in the stomach. Antacids not only curb the secretion of actual acid in the stomach, but prevent further stomach acid secretion. It is the latter that initiates a relief sensation after ingestion of antacids, which reduces villi functions on the stomach mucosa, resulting in *mucosal atrophy*, which may evolve into *atrophic gastritis*, a gathering place of dangerous bacteria like the Helicobacter pylon (H. pylon); the further evolution of *atrophic gastritis* is *stomach cancer.*[26]

---

[25]   The Enzyme Factor: Hiromi Shinya, MD, 2011
[26]   The Enzyme Factor: op. cit.

Digestion is a sequential process and occurs as eaten foods are dissolved and chemically transformed for cell absorption. Foods upstream of the alimentary canal need to adequately melt before they can pass through the intestinal wall. Ingested foods that take too long for digestion to take place may become fermented and hence toxic for the body, infecting the bloodstream with toxic wastes. Foods that are decomposed in the gut create poisonous chemicals that are so toxic that the body looks for ways to expel them out instantly.[27] Toxic chemicals or *indicans* can result from constipation and cause bowel irritation; their presence is an indication that proteins have not been well assimilated. The body may rid itself of *indicans* or toxic wastes through the eliminative channels, while others remain in the bloodstream and are likely to cause inflammatory problems—unless the liver expels them out.

Today consumers are seeking foods with a longer shelf life. This strong desire has fostered in many individuals a dependency for industrial foods, where enzymes have been destroyed through the refinement process. Food preparation, irradiation, and canning are some other methods by which foods are processed. In some cases, foods are even artificially grown to purposely lack enzymes.

Enzymes are a type of proteins or bonded amino acids that cells generate to accelerate chemical reactions. Scientists conveniently refer to them as catalysts since their chemical actions on other substances preserve their own state or status. Other reactants participate in the process, but in greater amounts. An enzyme is not automatically active. The protein constituent of the enzyme, apoenzyme, needs to be tightly connected to its cofactor known to be the prosthetic group in order to effectively function and trigger this dynamic.

Around the 1970s, Americans began to see that medications and surgeries do not always promote healing. As a result, patients were requesting from physicians, services that they were not trained to provide. By 1994, the number of patients who had sought alternative

---

[27] Enzymes—The Key to Health—Volume 1—The Fundamentals by Howard F. Loomis, Jr., D.C., F.I.A.C.A.

treatment was likely to be thirty to forty percent of the sick people. A study conducted around that time displayed people's willingness to pay out-of-pocket for their own care whenever necessary.

Contributing Factors to Obesity

Meanwhile, various debates and discussions on non-prescription and prescription drugs, trans-fats including hydrogenated oil, and artificial sweeteners have revealed that they get stored in the liver and lower the body metabolism. Cold water drinks, high refined food intake, missing morning breakfast, air conditioning use, muscle mass loss, and nutritional deficiencies (lack of vitamins, minerals, and amino acids) can deeply impact metabolism as well.[28] A properly functioning metabolism favors easy breathing, normal blood circulation, stable body temperature, proper digestion of food and nutrients, timely elimination of waste through urine and feces, and proper function of the brain and nerves, and so on.

The Lure of Gain

Few people know that laboratories spend their time changing the concept of disease and reshaping the public perception of disease.[29] The drug industry invents diseases in order to sell more drugs. Leading experts in the medical world in the United States, Australia and France, are attacking the reshaping of the concept of diseases. According to Dr Bruno Toussaint, laboratories would just gather some elements of diseases or disorders that some people are dealing with to transform them into serious diseases that affect many people.[30]

Professor Philippe Even, director of the Institute Necker in Paris, felt the same way when he said, "the drug industry expands its market and the perimeter of each disease to compensate for failure to patent new drugs." Professor Even added that "treating

---

[28] The Weight Loss Cure by Kevin Trudeau—2007
[29] Ray MOYNIHAN, Investigation Specialist in the British Medical Journal on the Daily Practices of Pharmaceutical Firms
[30] Director of the magazine PRESCRIBE, a totally independent magazine of the pharmaceutical industry

diabetes, high blood pressure, cholesterol and abdominal fat on the basis of the metabolic syndrome to someone who may have only the beginnings of one of them is a scam." He even suggested that this syndrome be banned from medical terminology.

A Canadian study conducted in 52 countries and in over 200 hospitals over five continents, and which involved 27,000 people, reports that the metabolic syndrome is an invented disease, wrongly claimed to be associated with diabetes, cholesterol, hypertension and abdominal fat.[31] The belly syndrome is a metabolic or scientific puffery.[32]

Medical evidence indicates that the Mediator diabetes drug, internationally marketed as Benfluorex, was a drug officially designed to lower blood sugar. Nevertheless, it has been proven to cause pulmonary hypertension leading to shortness of breath.[33] According to Professor Andre Grimaldi, a diabetes specialist at the Pitié Salpétrière Hospital in France, the scientific community has never recognized this drug as an anti-diabetic.

Critics of Professor Jean-Paul Giroud[34] go in the same direction. To him, indeed, the effectiveness of Mediator has never been shown to exist in studies conducted by the Laboratories Servier. Moreover, Professor Philippe Even, chairman of the Necker Institute, claimed that Mediator was presented as an amphetamine in an international congress six years before it was marketed. The allusion to amphetamine-like properties is not even written in the record of the drug.

In contrast, a study conducted in 1995[35] revealed that the risk of developing pulmonary hypertension is much higher with Isomeride than with Benfluorex (Mediator). Similar to Isomeride, whose

---

[31] Dr. Andrew MENTE, University MC MASTER
[32] The doctors of the journal PRESCRIBE in 2006
[33] Dr. Irene Frachon, author of "Mediator 150mg—How many deaths?", published in 2010
[34] Author of non-prescription medicines released in 05/2011
[35] Professor Lucien Abenhaim conducted the search, and the search results were published in the New England Journal of Medicine in 1995

marketing has been prohibited, Mediator releases norfenfuramine in the body, a substance potentially dangerous and harmful to health.

Mediator is known as one of the amphetamines or appetite suppressants. France banned all amphetamines in 1998 but not Mediator. Mediator, being an anorectic and weight reducer, indirectly reduces the level of glucose in the blood. One of the known side effects of Mediator (Benfluorex) is shortness of breath due to valvular disease,[36] characterized by thickening of the heart valves. Indeed, in a normal body the valves open and close quickly, while in valvulopathy, the thickened valves cause breathlessness in the patient even with the least physical effort.

A World Frighteningly Toxic

Studies have shown that both non-prescription and prescription drugs, lack of iodine and nutrients, and the presence of fluorine in toothpaste, drinking and bathing water, each have a negative bearing on thyroid dysfunction. Artificial substances, for example aspartame, are added to foods and drinks with the intent to enhance taste but instead produce various disorders including thyroid dysfunction. Indeed, the symptoms that aspartame can generate are legion. They vary from seizures, brain tumors, and hardening of the synovial fluid, coma, and even can lead to death.

Aspartame acts together with ingested drugs to damage the mitochondria and therefore accelerate memory debility. The mitochondria are minor components in a cell that facilitate the conversion of food into energy. Aspartame also works together with insulin to cause harmful effects to the retina of the eyes and trigger so-called diabetic retinopathy. So it is not diabetes that causes retinopathy, it is not diabetes that destroys the optic nerves and causes blindness, it is aspartame in most cases, according to a study Dr. Betty Martini cited.[37]

---

[36]   Dr. Chiche, a cardiologist at Marseille in France
[37]   Blood Sugar Control Linked to Memory Decline, posted on January 6, 2009, by Dr. Betty Martini

Scientific studies have proven that aspartame flows to the liver after ingestion and some transition time in the intestine. The liver transforms this substance into aspartic acid, methanol, and phenylalanine. The transformation requires a lot of energy from the liver cells which may become overworked in the process, and so lose their ability to burn fats and carry out necessary metabolic activities. Consequently, fats can start building up in the liver cells. As the storage time for aspartame is prolonged, the blood sugar level may become unstable and create a craving for sugar. Many diabetic patients have gone through a craving desire for carbohydrates, while others have experienced insulin resistance after ingestion of food or drink that contained aspartame.[38]

Dr. Betty Martini claimed that sugar has been blamed for causing diabetes when the most usual cause of the ailment is aspartame and MSG. Indeed, Type-II diabetes epidemic may have multiple causes, but for Dr. Ralph Walton as quoted by Dr. Martini, aspartame is the main cause of Type-II diabetes development.

The Dentate Gyrus

Aspartame can cause a sudden moderate blood sugar elevation in some people, or an extreme blood sugar elevation in others. In either case, this additive is known to have an effect on the dentate gyrus, which is an internal area of the brain to a composite structure in the medial temporal lobe of the brain known as the hippocampus which is critical to new memory formation and other bodily functions. A study involving magnetic resonance imagery has revealed a relationship between blood glucose elevation and a reduction of blood flow in the dentate gyrus. Dr. Roni Caryn Rabin quoted a study that found a link between Type-II diabetes and the dentate gyrus.

In an article, entitled, "Adverse Effects of Aspartame," Dr. Martini reported the results of an experiment conducted on 551 individuals and has classified the adverse effects of aspartame as being both psychiatric and psychological. Most of the individuals

---

[38]   The Molecular Holocaust of Aspartame, by Dr. Bill Deagle, MD

dealing with these effects of aspartame experienced multiple symptoms, ranging from headache, dizziness, unsteadiness, or both, confusion or memory loss or both, severe drowsiness and sleepiness, paresthesias (pins and needles or numbness of the limbs), convulsions (epileptic attacks), severe slurring of speech, severe tremors, severe hyperactivity and restless legs, extreme irritability, and so on.

Why our Organs are Usually Clogged?

Non-prescription and prescription drugs and food consumption devoid of fiber and digestive enzymes can all contribute to a clogged colon. A clogged or congested colon usually triggers constipation. Constipation exists when all the bowel movements for any given day does not eliminate waste from all the foods that have been eaten within the previous 17 to 24 hours.

Lack of water or water absorption may also be responsible for a clogged colon, which can slow down the digestive process, which in turn lessens the metabolism and eventually increases fat buildup. Water is one of four basic nutrients required for the whole organism.[39] Without water, biochemical activities are disturbed when they are not compromised. Water insufficiency or improper fluid distribution can lead to all sorts of diseases known to man. Therefore, diabetes is no exception. But most people are unaware that they are dehydrated. They do not even know that a low metabolism can be the result of dehydration. Kevin Trudeau, the author of The Weight Loss Cure, wrote "it is common to find in autopsies thirty pounds of undigested fecal matter in people's colon."

The colon has two sets of bacteria; one of which is detrimental to the body's biochemical activities. Antibiotics favor the unrestrained growth of the damaging ones, among them the Candida yeast, which may bring about a craving state of mind for bread, pasta, cheese, and sugar or the like. Candida can turn into fungus over time and spread throughout the body.

---

[39] Prescription for Nutritional Healing, Fifth Edition, by Phyllis A. Balch, CNC—2010

A sluggish colon and/or liver, stress, chemical additives in foods, fluorine and chlorine in drinking and bathing water, and the application of cosmetics and lotions on skin may all result in weight gain due to hormone imbalances. In excess, weight can cause humans to experience environmental and food allergies as a result of poor circulation, parasites, or heavy metal toxicity. Weight gain can also cause humans to develop insulin intolerance, which in turn can be caused by consumption of high fructose corn syrup, artificial sweeteners, nutritional deficiencies, Candida overgrowth, prescriptions and non-prescription drugs, food additives, and conditions like a clogged liver and colon. Insulin intolerance or insulin resistance occurs when body cells resist glucose assimilation.

In addition, heavy metals which include mercury from amalgam fillings can clog the liver and colon and slow down the circulation process. Poor circulation lowers the metabolism; this reduction in the metabolism often originates from clogged arteries, which in turn can be caused by fats and/or manmade trans-fats, cow injections, growth hormones in meat and drugs, mineral deficiencies, heavy toxicity, homogenized dairy products, and chlorine in water, etc. A clogged lymphatic system also triggers faulty metabolism, which may be associated with improper nutrition. Faulty metabolism prevents bone nutrition, deprives children of sleep, and causes tonsillitis and enlargement of cervical glands, which can lead to bronchitis and pneumonia. Faulty metabolism may also contribute to the softness and fatness of muscles.

The body needs an extra basic element known as polyunsaturated fatty acids, examples of which are Omega 3 and Omega 6. The body does not synthesize these fatty acids. Therefore they are essential, and have to be ingested from dietary sources. They are used to manufacture cell membranes, brain tissues, hormones and other chemicals, and to disseminate certain vitamins A, D, E and K.[40]

---

[40] Prescription for Nutritional Healing, Fifth Edition, by Phyllis A. Balch, CNC—2010

Many consumer foods are so high in calories that the body cannot even burn off the excess. In despair, the body converts those calories into fats and stores them in the body, which in the long run is a potential for weight gain and obesity. The body needs to burn calories efficiently in order to keep the body weight under control, and eventually prevent diseases, such as diabetes.

Our Future Food and Health

It is customary to hear "marketing experts" say that canned and jarred foods are pasteurized for the safety of forthcoming consumers. To be pasteurized, these foods have been heated to 180 degrees for 30 minutes. As in the microwave oven, this process destroys most if not all of the digestive enzymes in the foods. Enzyme deficiencies can result in gas, bloating, constipation, and a slow digestion. On the other hand, foods marketed in the United States, fruits and vegetables for instance, are genetically modified and gassed during the ripping process, which devoid them of enzymes. The body senses these foods as invaders, able to disrupt the body chemistry and deplete enzymes in the body. Hence, strain is put on the pancreas to secrete greater amounts of enzymes than normal, exhausting the pancreas.

The over-reliance on chemical fertilizers for about half a century has helped start an agricultural revolution at the expense of consumers. Pesticides, herbicides, and fungicides necessary for mass production have adverse effects on foods. They are full of chemicals, carcinogenic for the most part and have caused the degradation of taste in fruits and vegetables. These chemicals also contribute to soil depletion. Fertilizers can reduce the phosphorus content of a fruit, and the nitrogen in a chemical fertilizer can interfere with the ability of a plant to synthesize vitamin C. In other words, chemical fertilizers promote dangerous chemical reactions in nature and can result in harm to the human body.

The Reality of an Ongoing Crisis

Since 1963, the tomato has lost 30.7 percent of its vitamin A, 16.9 percent of its vitamin C, 61.5 percent of calcium and 9 percent of potassium. The reason is that fruits and vegetables are soaked in chlorine, undergo chamber maturation, gassing, injection of a dye, etc. Broccoli, often considered the symbol of healthy eating, has lost in the last half century over 60 percent of its calcium content and more than a third of its iron. Since 1936, spinach has lost 96 percent of its copper, 53 percent of its potassium, 70 percent of its phosphorus and 60 percent of its iron.[41]

A 1992 United Nations conference on Environment and Development in Rio de Janeiro, Brazil, highlighted other alarming findings. It was reported that the European agricultural lands lost up to 72 percent of their fertility and mineral content, while for the United States, the figure would reach this level of concern at 85 percent. This mineral deficiency, detrimental to good fertility, could reach the 100 percent level if one considers the large U.S. farms polluted due to massive fertilizer use.[42]

In addition, fruits and vegetables produced in the United States are dowsed in "heavily chlorinated water and highly irradiated." Chlorine alone can disturb the thyroid gland production and trigger low metabolism in the body. A common food additive or "excito toxin" called monosodium glutamate (MSG), is ordinarily used as a flavor enhancer and displayed on food labels.

The Evils of our Food

Flavor enhancers in our foods are manmade chemicals combined to create a symphony of taste. Natural flavors, which come from nature, do not necessarily mean what the labels imply. The food industry has intensified ingredients in a package, jar, can, with combinations of fats, sugar, and salt.

A former head of the US Food Drug Administration, David A. Kessler, M.D., once said, "The artificial flavors are so stimulating that they hijack our brain." He even believes that the flavorists are

---

[41] Toxic Food by William Reymond—2007
[42] Toxic Food, op. cit.

accomplices, i.e. hired guns of the flavor industry.[43] He retreated thereafter when he said that the flavor industry did not make use of artificial flavors on purpose, but built up strategies over time based on people's expectations. Nonetheless, Robert Pellegrino admits that they are simply trying to create irresistible and memorable tastes so that consumers can make repeat purchases.[44]

Sometimes dangerous ingredients printed on the packaging of food labels are unreadable because they are written in very small characters. Juices, sodas, yogurts, candy, chewing gum, lollipops, and most vitamin supplements are full of additives. The toxic aspartame has been marketed under different names, such as NutraSweet, Equal, Equal-Measure, Indulge, Spoonful, Canderel, E951, etc.[45]

Curiously, aspartame is hidden in more than 600 drugs and more than 6000 food products.[46] It has been said that young consumers of this toxic ingredient display, in general, the following symptoms: dark circles under the eyes, headaches, sleep disorders, skin problems, various allergies, repetitive infections (such as bronchitis), weight gain, anorexia or bulimia, back pain and/or knee pain (sometimes in the wrists), tremor of the legs, hair loss, depression, unexplained temper tantrums, learning delays, seizures, decreased number of platelets in the blood, spots to the brain, brain tumors, etc.

The Discovery of Aspartame

An American chemist at the GD Searle Company, James Schlatter, was conducting an experiment in 1965 on an anti-ulcer drug when he discovered Aspartame. Schlatter was the first to observe the deleterious effects of aspartame on the human body. Curiously, this substance, one of the most dangerous on the market,

---

[43] The End of Overeating: Taking Control of the Insatiable American Appetite by David A. Kessler, 2010

[44] Robert Pellegrino, the Executive Vice-President of Global Strategy and Business Development at Givaudan, the global leader in the flavor industry

[45] Additifs Alimentaires by Corinne Gouget—2010

[46] Additifs Alimentaires, op. cit.

is the additive of choice in children's vitamins and in chewing gum. It can turn on attention deficit disorder with or without genetic predispositions, as well as other conditions requiring psychiatric care, such as manic depression. Furthermore, aspartame interacts poorly with antidepressants. Too much aspartame in the brain can damage neurons and promote excess calcium in the cells.

Dr. Baret of the Dominican Republic conducted an experiment on 360 children, to whom he offered beverages that contain aspartame. He observed, after a while, significant changes in their behavior, so he decided not to continue feeding them the product containing aspartame. [47]

So far no researchers have noticed the presence of ethanol in aspartame,[48] but generally fruit juices and alcohol contain some methanol, which requires ethanol as an antidote to balance out the methanol toxicity. Folic acid can protect against methanol poisoning as it can accelerate the conversion of formic acid into carbon dioxide and water. The development of chronic methanol indigestion may come from folic acid deficiency.

Research has shown that a molecule of aspartame contains 40 percent aspartic acid, 10 percent methyl ester, and 50 percent phenylalanine. Phenylalanine has been identified as a neurotoxin and has a direct impact on the brain, as it depletes serotonin. Serotonin acts as neurotransmitter to regulate certain body functions, such as sleep, stress, mood, and behavior. Its depletion can therefore trigger manic depression or bipolar, suicidal tendency, mood swings, hallucinations, insomnia, panic attacks, etc. Aspartame is capable of protecting living tissues while harming the deoxyribonucleic acid (DNA). Aspartic acid is an amino acid resembling a neurotransmitter that transmits (in the brain) information from neuron to neuron. Phenylalanine and aspartic acid do not go through the metabolism which occurs in normal foods,

---

[47] Dr. Betty Martini, April 22, 2011
[48] Emerging Facts About Aspartame by Dr. J Barua and Dr. Al Bal, posted online on March 19, 2007

where food proteins in general are progressively broken down as the amino acids are gradually absorbed.

Proteins represent an additional basic element as vital to the body as water, carbohydrates, and fats. They can be obtained from plants or animals. Smart consumers need to make a wise choice because animals in the United States (including cows) are injected with antibiotics and hormones. Consumers with robust appetites for meat and milk ingest antibiotics and hormone residues that have toxic effects on the body. Furthermore, antibiotics can prevent the absorption of vitamin K, needed for bone integrity and the avoidance of blood clot formation. One of the direct effects of ingested hormones is weight gain, which frequently leads to obesity, creating a sympathetic environment for the development of diabetes, due to a metabolic disorder.

Dr. Juan Manuel Aparicio, geneticist and pediatrician at the Nino Poblano Hospital in Mexico, in an article published on October 17, 2009, presented the results of his study. He claimed that food containing aspartame can be the foundation of over 200 diseases, which may be characterized by a general state of fatigue, brain tumors, as well as osteoarthritis, multiple sclerosis, cerebral hemorrhage, thyroid problems, and bulimia, etc.

Some babies developed tumors at birth including brain cancer because their mother had absorbed during pregnancy products intensified with aspartame. Highly carcinogenic, aspartame had damaged the nervous and immune systems of the children, and suppressed the production of DNA (deoxyribonucleic acid) that controls our cell activities.

Simple and Complex Carbohydrates

Carbohydrates are one of the four basic elements critical for energy creation.[49] There are two kinds of carbohydrates: simple and complex carbohydrates. Simple carbohydrates are better known for their starchy substance, while complex carbohydrates are abundant

---

[49] Prescription for Nutritional Healing, Fifth Edition, by Phyllis A. Balch, CNC—2010

in fiber. Fiber is beneficial as it absorbs toxins, fats and sugar that can be in excess.

The Glycemic Index

Foods loaded with high glycemic values are referred to as high carbohydrates; others loaded with low glycemic values are referred to as low carbohydrates. The glycemic index is intended as a means to manage carbohydrate consumption. It sets the degree of absorption of sugar for simple and complex carbohydrates, as it allows people to keep track of possible glucose elevation in the bloodstream. The transformation time into glucose is inferior for low or complex carbohydrate foods, and superior for high or simple carbohydrate foods, which means that the latter enter the bloodstream faster and tend to activate insulin production.

Dr. David J. Jenkins was very concerned about abnormal sugar elevation occurring mostly after food consumption. He established, alongside colleagues, a tool that exhibits the glycemic value of most common foods in order to determine the timing for simple or complex carbohydrates to get metabolized into glucose and enter the bloodstream.

The idea behind the glycemic index is that food loaded with a high glycemic value may quickly elevate the blood sugar to a level that is intolerable by the human body, while a food with a low glycemic value is expected to slowly and moderately elevate the blood sugar and maintain it at a level that the human body can control. As time goes by the moderately increased glucose should go down and stabilize itself at the optimal level. An elevated blood sugar is viewed as a glucose imbalance, which may trigger the production of more insulin to help drive the glucose into the cells so it can be transformed into energy. Any extra glucose that is let out in the bloodstream can be rescued by the liver and the body muscles.

Diabetics use a meter reader that allows them to monitor their level of glycaemia. The glycemic index does not appear to be a universal tool for glycemic evaluation. Through the means of Applied Kinesiology, it has been found that the glycemic value of a food may vary from one diabetic to another. The glycemic index seems to have limitations in assessing the glycemic value of foods, and thus can be counter-productive. This tells people that different diabetics have different glycemic tolerance levels.

What is Diabetes, and What is Diabetes Mellitus?

Diabetes is mainly known to be a disease of the pancreas, characterized by blood sugar elevation beyond glycemic control. It is also known as a "gender-neutral disease" as it affects both men and women. The word diabetes came from the Greek word *diabaínein* that literally means "passing through," or "siphon", to refer to frequent urination once a diabetic condition exists. Typically the Latin term "mellitus," which means "honey sweet", is associated with the word diabetes to refer to the glucose lost in the urine. Diabetes is therefore an ailment that results from the body's failure to properly metabolize its glucose.

Orthodox medicine considers someone to be pre-diabetic once the blood glucose level falls between 100-125 mg/dl before meals and between 140-190 mg/dl two hours after meals. Likewise, orthodox medicine considers anybody with a blood glucose level attaining 126 mg/dl or more or a blood sugar level of more than 200, two hours after meals, to be diabetic.[50]

Muscles and tissues convert food ingestion into glucose for its assimilation. This glucose will then be metabolized in the body cells if there is no resistance to its attempt to enter cells. A bunch of cells known as The Islets of Langerhans are scattered throughout the pancreas to manufacture the hormone called insulin. The beta cells of the pancreas are responsible for releasing enough of this hormone to regulate the glucose in the bloodstream, and for routing it towards most of the billions of body cells. Hunger and satiety may then result from insulin stimulation of centers in the hypothalamus of the brain.[51]

---

[50] The Everything Guide to Managing and Reversing Pre-Diabetes by Gretchen Scalpi, RD, RCD, CDE

[51] Diabetes Solution, The Complete Guide to Achieving Normal Blood Sugars, by Richard K. Bernstein, MD—2007

As a matter of fact, the insulin hormone transforms glucose and fatty acids in the blood into fats. Fat cells store these fats for later use. According to Dr. Bernstein, insulin is an anabolic substance, vital for many tissue and organ development. In excess, insulin can cause the development of needless body fat and growth of cells that line the blood vessels. This substance helps regulate, or counter regulate, other hormones in the body. It regulates the liver and muscles and directs them to manufacture and store glycogen to maintain the narrow range of normal levels of glucose in the blood. Glycogen is known as a starchy substance the body uses when the blood sugar falls too low."[52]

What is Type-I Diabetes?

Diabetes can have a heredity component. Lots of people have relatives, a brother or a sister, and sometimes one or both parents and perhaps a child diagnosed with diabetes. According to Dr. Neal Barnard (2007), when the white blood cells of the body's immune system damage the pancreas so much that it can no longer produce insulin, that results in Type-I diabetes. But he does not believe that Type-I diabetes is exclusively a genetic disease. He believes it could be triggered by 'something' in the child's early environment. In fact, certain infants born with a genetic predisposition to develop diabetes never do so. In the case of twins, however, one of them may have Type-I diabetes while the other has less than a 40 percent chance of developing it.[53]

Research results indicate that Type-I diabetes is the consequence of the destruction of the insulin producing cells, the beta cells, due to immune attacks. This creates a craving for more insulin, which can only be satisfied through general injections, in order to respond to the excess of glucose in the bloodstream. Why does the body immune system attack the pancreatic beta cells in this manner?

---

[52] Diabetes Solution, The Complete Guide to Achieving Normal Blood Sugars, by Richard K. Bernstein, MD—2007

[53] The Scientifically Proven System for Reversing Diabetes Without Drugs by Dr. Neal D. Barnard, M.D.—2007

The body immune system is not designed to embark on any actions against any body parts;[54] it is designed to show aggression to foreign invaders. For some reasons, however, the body immune system may think that an invading bacteria or germ is around or in the beta cells and start engulfing it, and, in the process, damages or destroys the beta cells. The beta cells can be viewed as "innocent spectators" that may get injured in a sudden attack.

Besides friendly bacteria, harmful and toxic bacteria are present in the intestine. These damaging bacteria generate toxins and may as well trigger immune responses. In case of an immune attack to eliminate foreign invaders, further damages can occur and cause many ailments, such as Crohn's disease and celiac disease, etc.

Bifidobacteria can produce digestive enzymes like lysozyme and phosphate, B-vitamin and folic acid, speed up immune attacks against tremor cells, assist in the absorption of calcium and magnesium, alter the growth of destructive bacteria, crowd out dangerous toxin-generating germs, and decelerate the production of damaging protein breakdown products.[55]

Daily ingestion of Bifidophilus Flora Force and Probiotic Eleven is recommended to prevent the proliferation of antagonistic bacteria. Probiotic effectiveness has been proven, as the most prevailing probiotic, fructooligosaccharide, also known as oligofructose, is involved in about three hundred enzyme reactions. Some of these reactions include maintaining blood sugar at the optimum level, improving liver function and fostering calcium and magnesium absorption.

How does the Type-II diabetes differ from the Type-I diabetes?

According to the American Diabetes Association, 90 to 95 percent of people diagnosed with diabetes are Type-II diabetes, formerly called adult-onset diabetes or non-insulin-dependent diabetes. It occurs when glucose is elevated in the bloodstream

---

[54] Dr. Rallie McAllister, M.D. Nature's Sunshine 2008 National Convention
[55] ANDRESCOINCORPORATED—2005

beyond the optimal level and the pancreas has been unable to meet its obligation for more insulin.

Martin-Gronert and Ozanne[56] conducted a study on whether Type-II diabetes can be associated with birth weight. Sixty-four year old adult-men were part of the study. The results showed that the risk of developing Type-II diabetes was six times greater for those with a lower birth weight than for those with an elevated birth weight. This study was repeated worldwide over forty different populations. It produced the same results.

Martin-Gronert and Ozanne observed similar relationships between birth weight and insulin resistance. This statement seems to establish a link between low weight at birth and a risk for insulin resistance. However, since the fact that the experimental group was partly composed of people who were born with maternal obesity, birth weight should not be used as a basis to explain insulin resistance, as it would be biased. Further studies are therefore needed in order to arrive at a more precise conclusion.

Is Fighting Diabetes a Losing Battle?

Diabetes is increasing in the United States, with the number of people diagnosed with Type-II diabetes in 2001 reached sixteen million. This figure is increasing by an additional 800,000 cases per year.[57] Yale University revealed in a study that 25 percent of obese teenagers are Type-II diabetes. Overall, about 80 percent of Type-II diabetics are overweight or obese. Obese people in general are insulin resistant; that is, the ability of the insulin to transport glucose in body cells is diminished as blood sugar rises.

Most people with Type-II diabetes still produce insulin, but their cells refrain from accepting it, and the body is therefore forced to maintain the production of insulin to overcome the resistance.[58] Failure to surmount the resistance may result in glucose buildup in

---

[56] The Journal of Nutrition, 2010
[57] The Journal of Nutrition by Samuel T. Nadler and Alan D. Attie, 2001
[58] The Scientifically Proven System for Reversing Diabetes Without Drugs by Dr. Neal D. Barnard, M.D.

the bloodstream. "Diabetes drugs work to counteract this problem. Some make your cells more responsive to insulin. Others cause your pancreas to release more insulin into the bloodstream or block your liver from sending extra glucose into the blood."[59] An enzyme so important for diabetic patients, CoQ10 for heart attack prevention, may be destroyed in the process. Looking forward, blood glucose concentration can damage arteries, nerves, blood vessels of the eyes, kidneys, and other body parts.

What is Special about Gestational Diabetes?

Gestational diabetes is a form of diabetes that occurs solely during pregnancy as either Type-II diabetes or as a sign of imminent Type-II diabetes. Otherwise, it soon ceases to exist. In gestational diabetes, the pancreatic production of insulin does not end but body cells counteract its actions. Orthodox medicine believes that a combination of medications and lifestyle changes can maintain glycemic levels close to the non-diabetic range.

The safeness of sugar, alcohols, and nonnutritive sweetness for diabetics are part of the limits and standards the Food and Drug Administration and the American Diabetes Association[60] have set respectively for medical care with regard to diabetics. In contrast, drinking alcohol destroys cells; even wine destroys cells. But while wine has some chemicals that destroy cells, it also has nutrients that extend the life of some cells.

Proteins, collagen, and enzymes in an unbalanced blood sugar can damage cellular DNA and accelerate aging. Statistics from insurance companies have shown that 29-year-old diabetics have a life expectancy of 16 years less than that of non-diabetics, 39-year-old diabetics have a life expectancy of 11 years under the expected life of non-diabetics, and 49-year-old diabetics have expected life duration of 10 years less than that of non-diabetics. Normally a shorter lifespan is anticipated for non-diabetics with unstable blood glucose.

---

[59]   The Scientifically Proven System for Reversing Diabetes Without Drugs by Dr. Neal D. Barnard, M.D.
[60]   The American Diabetes Association, 2008

Excess glucose may stimulate the production of proteins that are damaged by sugar. These types of proteins are called glycated proteins, and can react to oxygen in order to generate superoxide free radicals, which can degrade collagen, the body structural matrix, and create advanced glycation end products that cause aging. Glycated proteins can transform themselves into hydrogen peroxide and hydroxyl radicals, two free radicals[61] that are more powerful than superoxide, and likely to cause much destruction to the proteins of human tissues, organs, immune system and muscles.

In excess, glucose can alter the kidneys and trigger cardiovascular disease and arteriosclerosis. Diabetics need low glycemic foods, such as dried apricot, buckwheat, fructose, brown rice, barley, magnesium, and so on. Magnesium depletion, which is a causative factor to aging, is a contributor to angina, arteriosclerosis, depression, cardiac arrhythmia, high blood pressure and diabetes. Angina is a condition involving severe chest pains due to lack of blood circulation in the heart.

The Very Tip of a Much More Dangerous Iceberg

The American Diabetes Association has discouraged the use of chromium for diabetics on the basis of there being no conclusive substantiation. Through my practices and those of colleagues in the health field, Applied Kinesiology has repeatedly demonstrated that chromium is the key element to combat pancreatic weakness. Chromium works very well on the pancreas to address any deficiencies in chromium or insulin production. Exclusive to my practices, and again thanks to Applied Kinesiology, sugar cane is often recommended for people experiencing diabetes and planning their vacations either in the Caribbean or in Africa where they can easily have access to it.

The American Diabetes Association is doubtful about the effectiveness of food supplements just as with vitamins E, vitamin C for lack of convincing evidence on long-term safety. It

---

[61] Free radicals result from industrial fumes, toxic particles, toxins, and other pollutants, which can cause damages to liver, kidneys, etc.

therefore discouraged the use of daily supplementation. Vitamin E is an enhancer for proper functioning of muscle, blood and nerve cells. It also assists in the absorption of unsaturated fats, fights off stress, and assists in detoxification. It works on cell surfaces as antioxidants. A single vitamin E molecule can fight up to one thousand free radicals in the human body. Vitamin E improves tissues' ability to use oxygen, and is an immune enhancer.

As for vitamin E, vitamin C is beneficial for everyone, and any amount intake should be increased when dealing with stress and any pathology. Hoffer and Walker[62] have considered vitamin C as the safest nutrient known, and taken daily and in appropriate dose can remarkably free the body of side effects and toxicity.

Vitamin C participates in bone, teeth and cartilage building. It participates in the formation of white blood cells to ensure that the body is protected against infections, drug residues and toxic particles in the environment. It promotes growth, while preventing nutrients from being oxidized. Daily consumption of vitamin C shields the circulatory system from fat deposits.

Summary: In consideration, both prescription and nonprescription drugs, inflammatory foods, food additives such as aspartame and monosodium glutamate, taste enhancers and other food rations deficient in fiber and enzymes, all have a deleterious effect on metabolism and may therefore have hyperglycemic effects.

---

[62] Putting It All Together: The New Orthomolecular Nutrition by Abraham Hoffer, M.D., Ph.D & Morton Walker, D.P.M., 1996

CHAPTER 3

RESEARCH DESIGN

As already indicated, this study has examined the six research questions via the interviews of colleagues in the health field and through my personal experiences with my clients.

The Research and Deductive Methods

The research method uses inferential procedures so that the researcher may make inferences about a larger set of measurements called a population (Dr. Lyman Ott 1988). Four naturopathic doctors each with a minimum of ten years of experience formed the sample. The sample represents the entire New York City area, where these particular naturopathic doctors have their practices. For the purpose of this study, the New York City area comprises four boroughs: Manhattan, Bronx, Queens, and Brooklyn. I have excluded Staten Island, the more suburban borough of New York City. The rationale for the number of samples is that each of the four naturopathic practitioners has had experience with hundreds of diabetics. Therefore each response represents a minimum of one hundred clients.

The deductive method allows one to generate a theoretical framework to pinpoint my hypotheses. In this particular study, it allowed one to consider ingested ingredients of any kind that are hyperglycemic in their metabolic actions, such as drugs and non-prescription drugs, food additives like monosodium glutamate, flavor enhancers, etc. It also permitted enunciating working hypotheses, implementing a grid interview for data collection and assessment of these hypotheses by means of content analysis.

Procedures for Testing the Research Questions

The testing procedures first considered the independent variable (food consumption) and the dependent variable (diabetes). Since food consumption has become a health issue all over the world, I have set up a causal relationship between food consumption and obesity.

As stated in the research question, this study is seeking to determine among other things whether diabetes is a function of food consumption, $D = f(Fc)$. Which of the variables is a function of the other is determined by which variable is dependent on the other variable's data variations. In other words, the independent variable is the variable that acts on its own without anything affecting it, whereas the dependent variable changes according to the influence of the independent variable.

Along with the eventual existence of correlation between food consumption and diabetes, contingent factors (such as free radicals, stress, dehydration, and emotion) may further impact the results. Thus, I added other independent variables, such as heredity, the hepatic system, the glandular system, mineral and vitamin deficiencies, and the previously mentioned contingent factors. This has determined the type of questions generated in the grid interview.

A Comparative Research

I have reported here the experiences of colleagues with their diabetic clients within the New York City area. My knowledge and experiences with diabetic clients are implicit in this study. Therefore this research is to some extent a comparative research study.

I had anticipated correlations between the independent predictor variables[63] and the dependent variable.[64] For this reason, I turned the research questions into seven directional hypotheses that predict a

---

[63]   The independent variables are food consumption, heredity, the glandular system, the hepatic system, vitamin and mineral deficiencies, contingent factors, such as stress and emotion, dehydration, and free radicals.

[64]   The dependent variable is diabetes.

direct correlation between each of the independent variables and the dependent variable. Correlation statistics allow me to display how each of the independent variables is related or correlated to diabetes.

A Chain of Hypotheses

The overall research question is to determine whether diabetes is the final result of all the predictor independent variables: food consumption, heredity, the glandular system, the hepatic system, vitamin and/or mineral deficiencies, and contingent factors mentioned earlier.

The independent variables relate to each other in the sense that they may each act alone or concomitantly on the dependent variable, diabetes. I joined groups of specified independent variables with each other to eventually bring up links. In other words, I sought for thematic concomitants to identify the variables or factors always associated with diabetes and those acting alone. The design of this study is to test the following hypotheses, assuming that a high level of glucose in the blood is not necessarily associated with pancreatic malfunction:

Hypothesis 1: A level of glucose beyond the ideal can result from the exclusive action of ingested foods leading to obesity.

Hypothesis 2: A level of glucose beyond the ideal can result from hereditary factors, such as social frustrations and injustices, characterized by emotional stress, stored in the DNA of parents, grandparents, and great grandparents that they have passed on to their descendants.

Hypothesis 3: A level of glucose beyond the ideal can result from the concomitant action of ingested foods, dehydration, and hepatic dysfunction.

Hypothesis 4: A level of glucose beyond the ideal can result from the concomitant action of ingested foods, dehydration, and glandular dysfunction.

Hypothesis 5: A level of glucose beyond the ideal can result from the concomitant action of vitamin and/or mineral deficiencies.

Hypothesis 6: A level of glucose beyond the ideal can result from the concomitant action of ingested food and free radicals in the body.

Hypothesis 7: A level of glucose beyond the ideal can result from the concomitant action of ingested foods, dehydration, and the individual's inability to manage stressful and emotional situations.

Responses to open-ended questions asked during the interviews represent the investigative corpus. I tested the hypotheses and drew conclusions after a detailed analysis. A hypothesis is a tentative explanation of reality which highlights a cause and effect relationship between two or more variables.

Process of Data Collection

I utilized interviews as a means or technique for data collection, and questionnaires as support for proper questioning. To this account, I interviewed four naturopathic doctors and used a tape recorder to ensure the accuracy of their responses.

The Questionnaire

I wrote the questionnaire or interview grid in English and mostly integrated open-ended questions. Each question consists of only one issue at a time. Prospective respondents are Creole, French, and English speakers. As expected, the respondents, throughout the interviews answered in a mixture of languages but primarily in Creole and partially in English. I asked each respondent to add any further information that he or she felt was necessary. I pre-tested the questionnaire or interview grid before its use, although a pre-testing group appeared unnecessary since the above mentioned health practitioners are colleagues or colleagues of colleagues. I analyzed responses to open-ended questions and reported as acknowledged, along with personal comments or analyses wherever necessary.

A Practitioner-Oriented Research

Since this study is not patient-oriented, but a practitioner-oriented research, I encouraged respondents to offer any valuable information they have acquired through their practices. I integrated this information into the analyses of the results. I knew in advance the best time to telephone each prospective respondent to increase the likelihood for quality information.

The Required Time to Complete the Interviews

About two weeks were necessary for interview completion. For optimal data collection, I took into account the schedules of the prospective respondents for a given day or week and contingent factors, such as their mood during the interview.

I translated verbatim from the recorder responses to open-ended questions asked during the interviews. These responses make up the corpus used to test the hypotheses, a hypothesis being a temporary construction of reality. I constructed the coded information from the interview transcripts into ten manageable and pertinent categories; the size of each is dependent on the data collection format. I adjusted the categories to break off the overlapping information in the interview transcripts.

I examined these categories using content analysis. Content analysis allows researchers to count and determine the frequency of concepts or phrases or a text and to examine relationships among them. I also examined each concept within a category to first determine the frequency at which this concept appears in the text, taking into account whether its appearance is explicit or implicit, and whether respondents used synonyms and homonyms. The rationale for this is to make sure that each category accurately measures eventual links among variables.

In carrying out content analysis procedures, I found relationships between the independent variables as they acted concomitantly on the dependent variable: diabetes. In other words, I discovered thematic concomitants, that is to say, identifying variables or factors still associated by similarity to diabetes and variables that always act separately or in isolation. I tested the hypotheses one at a time in order to highlight the determinants of diabetes. To avoid biases, I tested the hypotheses from the recorded interview transcripts.

I analyzed the interview transcripts to highlight the presence and the frequency of specific terms or concepts. Frequency is counting the number of occurrences of an event. I color-coded terms or words with the highest frequency and I excluded prepositions and definite or indefinite articles. I based percentages and comparisons on the number of word or phrase occurrences, which resolve the direction and intensity of these words or phrases.

Summary: All in all, this practitioner-oriented research has utilized the deductive method as the general orientation. It also uses grid interviews for data collection and content analysis as a general procedure for setting categories and determining similarities and differences among them to test the hypotheses. The findings and analyses that follow form the overall outcomes that make up this study.

CHAPTER 4

ANALYSES OF FINDINGS

Four naturopathic doctors currently practicing Applied Kinesiology (AK) verbally responded to my interviews. Coders reduced their responses to "affirm" or "did not affirm" binary categories, adjusted to break off overlapping information in the interview transcripts. I tested the hypotheses using content analysis.

I conducted four different sets of interviews using the same grid interview to search for correlations based on collected information. The specific aim was to predict probabilities of affirmative responses towards the factors of diabetes by naturopathic doctors who practiced AK for at least ten years. This set of analyses reflects my past experiences with clients principally across New York City. I organized the results in the following sections.

Section I

The results of the responses unanimously voiced toward food consumption and obesity leading to diabetes. Strong evidence exists suggesting that the diet of obese people consists mainly of food and drink that may contain harmful additives.

It appears from the series of interviews conducted that diabetes has many causes, but foremost is obesity due to food consumption. Excessive carbohydrates can create sugar overloads in the bloodstream and increase the need for more insulin production. It is important to lower carbohydrate ingestion so the blood is not overloaded with sugar.

Hypothesis 1

Hypothesis 1: The first hypothesis linked the independent variable (exclusive action of ingested foods leading to obesity can result in an excessive level of glucose) to the dependent variable (diabetes). The four practicing naturopathic doctors unanimously affirmed this hypothesis (100 percent), but some included the harmful effects of malnutrition, dehydration, stress, and emotions on the human body. The fourth doctor interviewed did not give a strong affirmative response to stress-emotions as a cause of diabetes giving the ratio of affirmative to non-affirmative responses for stress-emotions as a causative factor of diabetes as 3:1.

The doctors divided their responses evenly 2:2 with stress-emotions as the main cause of diabetes. The ratio of affirmative to non-affirmative responses of malnutrition as being a cause of diabetes was split equally 2:2. The first doctor stated that the brain synchronizes little or no ingested foods. This made the ratio of stress-emotions to malnutrition to little or no synchronization of ingested foods by the brain as being the principal reason for diabetes as 2:1:1.

Some Type-II diabetics are dealing with an apparent complete pancreatic failure and so bear a resemblance to Type-I diabetes. The reason is that their diet consists mostly of refined foods, white sugar and white flour and the refining process produces depressed or totally depleted chromium retention. This forces the insulin-manufacturing organ to produce much more insulin—to no avail. Hence some Type-II diabetics become insulin dependent and are mistakenly re-diagnosed, by assimilation, as Type-I diabetes. Chromium may help diabetics of all types with the daily dose depending on the degree of damage to the pancreas. Pro pancreas, fiber, Blood Sugar Formula, exercise, and a healthy diet will be beneficial as well.

All adult Type-II diabetics should always be categorized as Type II, never de-classified and re-classified as Type I, regardless of the degree of insulin dependency.

Section II

One possible explanation for a link between heredity and diabetes is the following. The body has been unable to recognize chromium (heredity factor) and continuously expels it, which causes pancreatic failure. As the causes of diabetes are diverse, there are several competing notions about the development of this ailment. Moreover, there exist a glaring lack of explanations for the Type I diabetes. This book fills in some of the gaps of a major unsolved puzzle in the empirical medicine literature.

Most people believe descendants are likely to acquire any of the ailments of their ancestors. They fail to acknowledge that heredity or genes do not predestine anyone to disease (predestination); it may however determine the likely form of a disease (predisposition).[65] That is to say, certain people may be prone to asthma, others to diabetes based upon genetic predispositions. Most of them will never develop any of these ailments if they regularly cleanse their body and ingest consistently proper nutrition in their diet.

Hypothesis 2

The second hypothesis tested the independent variable (above optimum glucose levels can result from hereditary factors) and the dependent variable (diabetes). The four practicing doctors provided affirmative opinions. Two out of four or 50 percent confirmed that a damaged chromosome was a hereditary or historical factor, while the other 50 percent asserted that at birth the human body was unable to assimilate chromium. Needless to say, such a finding brings to light the causative hereditary factor of Type I diabetes.

Type-I diabetes concerns only children since only they can develop this type of diabetes and therefore are insulin dependent. Adults with the so-called Type-1 diabetes acquired it during childhood. It makes no sense, however, for children who are chromium deficient to have the diagnosis of Type-I diabetes solely due to their youthful age. The rationale is that their immune

---

[65] Your Health . . . Your Choice by Ted Morter, Jr., M.A.—2009

system normally is strong enough to prevent almost any diseases. Therefore, the idea that children with Type-I diabetes have complete pancreatic failure becomes biased and therefore misleading. What actually happens is that the body does not recognize chromium; any chromium arriving gets expelled because of a damaged chromosome. Without chromium, the pancreas cannot produce insulin and the body will not absorb chromium until restoration of the damaged chromosome.

Orthodox medicine does not believe Type-I diabetes is reversible because they have no idea that a damaged chromosome is fixable as in cases of arthritis where a damaged chromosome is also involved. Contrary to orthodox medicine, most AK practitioners know that Type-I diabetes is hereditary and genetic and therefore cannot develop during adulthood.

Many diabetics are insulin intolerant, which indicates that insulin production repeatedly fails to drive excess glucose into cell membranes for assimilation and conversion into energy to prevent fatigue, to gradually lower blood sugar levels in the bloodstream, and to decrease the need for more insulin ingestion. All of these can only be accomplished when chromium is present to accelerate the enzyme-like substance production known as the Glucose Tolerance Factor—GTF. In other words, chromium deficiency may decelerate this enzyme-like substance production causing a steady elevation in blood glucose leading to the so-called diabetes mellitus. Such a condition or phenomena is habitual in the United States since the "western diet is abundant in refined, chromium depleted carbohydrates," and American farms are deficient in chromium. Furthermore, tissue chromium is much less abundant in the American population than in Asian populations. Nevertheless, the body requires chromium to metabolize carbohydrates. Since chromium always competes with other metals (zinc as an example) for its absorption, only five to ten percent of ingested chromium is generally absorbed.

Section III

People, both in and outside the medical field, are frequently skeptical regarding the role the liver or hepatic system may play in diabetes, unless they have had adequate training and understanding about how the different body systems work and affect one another.

Hypothesis 3

The third hypothesis tested the independent variable (above optimum glucose levels can result from concomitant factors of ingested foods, dehydration, and hepatic dysfunctions) and the dependent variable (diabetes). The four practicing doctors all affirmed this hypothesis, but the third respondent did not explicitly mention whether the possibility of dehydration and hepatic dysfunction factors could be a cause of above optimum glucose levels, dropping the affirmation percentage to 3 out of 4, or 75 percent. Nevertheless, dehydration, a major stress producer, can alter the balance of cells, tissues, organs, endocrines, kidneys, amino acids, and the digestive system.[66] Furthermore, lack of body fluids negatively affects nutrient transport and lymph movements throughout the body.[67]

Some functions of the body seem to continue to be a mystery to most health professionals and even to some physicians. Orthodox medicine focuses on the pancreas to diagnose and remedy diabetes, but the pancreas could be a secondary reason. They believe Type-I diabetes is present when the cells of the Islets of Langerhans in the pancreas completely fail to produce insulin; they also believe Type-II diabetes (adult onset diabetes) is present when there is partial damage to the Islets of Langerhans cells. What they fail to acknowledge is that the pancreas may function properly even though there is blood sugar elevation. The escalation in blood glucose may be associated with the whole digestive system including a weak or overworked liver. Supplementation with milk thistle, dandelion, or liver cleanse formula can help unclogged the liver, prevent toxin accumulation in the bloodstream, and enhance enzyme secretion.

The digestive system is made up of several different organs. Even though each organ performs specific tasks in the body, the

---

[66]   The Body Talk System by John Veltheim, Module 2, Seventh Edition
[67]   See The Body Talk System, op. cit.

liver due to its many metabolic functions is considered to be the organizer of the digestive organs. Some traditions even consider the liver as the focal point of the soul.

Liver cells transport blood pouring in and around the liver to the vena cava, which flows into the heart. The gastrointestinal wall absorbs nutrients and the liver processes them for storage and future use.[68] The liver attaches all sugars that the intestine absorbs into glycogen,[69] a giant starch chain molecule. The rationale is that a healthy liver can absorb a large amount of sugar from the blood and transform it into glycogen, which can later be released in the bloodstream when sugar is needed. Doing so usually prevents the circulatory system from having an excess of sugar. Experiencing a rush of energy right after eating a candy bar may be an indication that the candy bar has a very large amount of sugar or that the liver is weak or overwhelmed.

A circulation full of sugar calls for more insulin production to lower the sugar in the bloodstream. Insulin makes the cell membranes permeable enough for easy access of sugar that has been in excess in the bloodstream. It may be that too much insulin has been released in the bloodstream, causing too much sugar to enter the cells, which brings down the blood sugar low enough to cause hypoglycemia.

Any sugar that has been accommodated into the cell membranes is stored as fats and remains as fats. A low glycogen in the liver can bring the blood sugar below the optimal level, and increase the desire for sweet foods. This would initiate a vicious cycle, meaning too much sweet food raises the blood sugar level, triggering a need for more insulin. More insulin production triggers a low blood sugar, which can cause a person to be craving again for sweet foods eventually leading that individual to be overweight.

The liver reassembles into proteins the amino acids that have been absorbed by the small intestine. Normally the liver transports

---

[68] Diet & Nutrition—A Holistic Approach—by Rudolf Ballentine, MD
[69] Glycogen is a huge storage molecule that is in some ways similar to starch

amino acids to the rest of the body so they can be transformed into proteins for cell nourishment. Albumin is the most important protein that is formed in the process. It clears fluid out of tissues by means of osmosis.[70] A lack of albumin in the blood may lead to fluid retention and swelling. As a result, the body cells can break down to the degree where they are unable to allow enough protein in the bloodstream to bring and keep albumin at the normal level. Maintaining the blood sugar at the optimal level is very important for body cell survival, especially brain and heart cells. The entire body, starting with the intellect, may suffer as a result of a liver dysfunction.

Section IV

While there is prior evidence about a causal link between the glandular system and diabetes, other characteristics of glandular effects are also noted.

Hypothesis 4

The fourth hypothesis tested the independent variable (above optimum glucose levels can result from naturally accompanying actions of ingested foods, dehydration, and glandular dysfunction) and the dependent variable (diabetes). The four respondents unanimously gave affirmative opinions giving them tied ranks of 4 out of 4 identical to hypotheses 1 and 2, even though one respondent provided an implied answer when this AK practitioner said that any weakness in a body system may add to an imbalance in another body system. In fact, the respondents affirmed that a weakness in the glandular system and/or a slowdown in organ functions can have negative effects on the digestive system that incorporates the pancreas.

Amino acids play an important role in the body. Therefore, amino acids that the body cannot synthesize necessitate ingestion from foods. Both synthesized and non-synthesized amino acids transform into proteins for muscle mass, skin, nails, hair renewal,

---

[70] Osmosis is the movement of molecules of water from a higher to a lower concentration.

and transport of molecules into cells. The pancreas can also change proteins into enzymes and insulin. Proteins are involved in the construction and repair of the body and may come from both vegetable and animal sources. In fact, green leafy vegetables contain complete proteins that are capable of operating with all the essential amino acids. Hyperglycemic individuals can benefit from a diet rich in vegetable proteins, because the release of these proteins into the bloodstream is so slow that insulin is not produced beyond necessity.

Animal proteins are not so adaptable to humans. Meats are full of antibiotics and growth hormones, and humans absorb their residues when consumed. Several diseases usually affect meat eaters, and most of these diseases are usually degenerative. The human stomach does not secrete enough hydrochloric acid to digest meat as compared to the feline and canine stomachs that produce twenty times more hydrochloric acid than that of humans.

Undigested meat may rot and fall into decay producing polyps, parasites, bacteria and toxins. The digestive system may absorb toxins and cover it with flesh causing one to become overweight leading straight to diabetes. The biologist, Charles Darwin, highlighted that the natural food for humans was vegetables. Undigested meat can cause swelling and become an inner lining of the digestive tract and, over time, become a black rubbery substance known as mucoid plaque.

The pancreas secretes three different enzymes that vary according to food ingestion. Different enzymes perform different activities. The body has an enzyme that aids in digesting carbohydrates, as well as an enzyme that acts on fats to prevent fat buildup and heart malfunction. Another enzyme breaks down proteins to avoid protein buildup and kidney failure. If the enzyme that regulates carbohydrates is not produced, the body may have difficulty metabolizing carbohydrates which can lead to blood glucose disorders.

Exocrine and endocrine glands secrete substances to meet the diverse needs of the human body. The exocrine glands have ducts for their secretions to pass through and get to the point where biochemical actions are most needed. The endocrine glands are not equipped with ducts, so they pour their secretions called hormones into the bloodstream through small vessels or capillaries. Some endocrine glands like the thyroid affect digestion, nutrition and weight gain. Being overweight can create an environment conducive to the developing of obesity and diabetes.

In fact, the body functions like an orchestra, where several musicians are playing a partition. If one of them plays the partition wrong, the entire partition is in question. Similarly, if a certain number of people living in a house made the decision to no longer communicate to each other, then everyone in the house will suffer. This analogy means that the body is a chain of organs that are supposed to communicate with each other. For example, the adrenal glands send signals to the pancreas ensuring that the blood sugar does not go beyond a certain level. Feelings of resentment may affect ovaries, kidneys, etc. to the point where the ovaries or kidneys can no longer communicate with each other. The body or body systems should guide healers when tests are performed. No matter how well we eat, whether we eat organic foods or not, if the body does not synchronize them (the complete system needs to be synchronized), health issues may arise; the integral system, not just the brain, always needs balance.

Complications and time constraints are possible obstacles when one examines an infant. In fact, diseases acquired from the mother that have damaging effects on the infant can desynchronize the child's body. For instance, normal expectations for asthma or cancer for a 5-year old are almost non-existent. However, the child may have inherited health conditions from the uterus or womb of the mother, if she had been exposed to chemicals or air pollution. The normal infant organism is usually strong and well balanced, and is not supposed to absorb defective materials such as aluminum from the mother.

A pregnant woman who develops a deep concern as to whether her fiancé will marry her may have already given ailments of worry to the fetus; this emotion can become so destructive that it affects the lungs, the adrenals, the heart, the nerves, the kidneys, etc. This active emotion may lead to inadequate supplement intake. The best decision would be to de-activate the emotion, then balance and rebuild the system. Humiliated people need to release the emotion associated with the humiliation, because certain organs and especially the kidneys may hold that humiliation as a negative emotion.

The thymus gland, responsible for muscular strength, produces hormones whose secretions contribute to electrical impulses that regulate heartbeats and biochemical activities in the entire body. Located behind the sternum bone, composed of lymphatic tissues, it plays a role in T-cell formation, which serves among other things the crucial purposes of the destruction of foreign invaders and cancer cell destruction.

The adrenal glands, located above the kidneys, produce adrenaline. This hormone, in carrying out its metabolic reactions, regulates blood pressure and blood glucose formulation at optimal levels. The adrenaline secretions may add to the elimination of inflammation in different body parts including the bronchi, thus preventing asthma from developing. Asthma manifests itself in the lungs and the respiratory system, but its root really comes from the adrenal glands. Nourishing the adrenals with Adrenal Support may help overcoming asthma.

Section V

This study clearly highlights the importance of proper nutrition. People with vitamin and/or mineral deficiencies are prone to develop multiple diseases including diabetes.

Hypothesis 5

The fifth hypothesis tested the independent variable (above ideal glucose levels can result from the naturally associated actions of vitamin and/or mineral deficiencies) and the dependent variable (diabetes). Four respondents gave affirmative opinions (100%), and all emphasized that vitamin and/or mineral deficiencies cause general weakness to the body.

Minerals combined with large protein molecules, also called **enzymes**, carry on their metabolic functions. In doing so, they sustain human life. Bones serve as calcium storage for later use. Gravity plays an important role in retaining calcium in the bone and in maintaining the overall skeletal system. Bedridden patients, newly accustomed to a sedentary life, may lose far more calcium than active patients, and elderly people are no exception. They are prone to osteoporosis[71] because many lack quality calcium intake: they no longer exercise and they are losing bone mass as they get older. At the same time, any excess calcium can become cumbersome and impede the assimilation of iron, manganese, and zinc.

Other types of minerals, zinc for example, are known as trace elements.[72] They ensure through chemical connections with carbon, nitrogen, oxygen and hydrogen, to help develop new compounds. Zinc facilitates the exhalation of carbon dioxide through the lungs, and like the other trace minerals, participates in the inner functioning of cells.

The common minerals that the body needs to properly function are magnesium, calcium, phosphorus, potassium, sodium, etc. Leafy green vegetables and sesame seeds are among the calcium-rich foods. One should ingest Sesame seeds in small quantities as their digestive transit time may be very lengthy.

Section VI

The results raise the possibility that free radicals can destroy the DNA within the cell causing the pancreas to become diseased as a result. They also show that free radical contributors including dehydration, medications, bacteria, fungi and parasites can trigger diabetes. Abnormalities in the spleen, liver, gall bladder, kidney, adrenal and thyroid glands are free radical supporters. Negative emotional stress, and undue pressure on the pancreas from the ribs including sources

---

[71] Softness of the bones, which is one of the signs of aging

[72] These trace elements are zinc, manganese, iodine, and arsenic.

that are accidental and shocks (emotional or physical), are also considered to be free radical contributors. Although these variables are positively correlated with diabetes, the coefficients are not large for any of them.

Hypothesis 6

The sixth hypothesis tested the independent variable (above ideal glucose levels can result from the naturally occurring action of ingested foods and free radicals and the dependent variable (diabetes). Three out of four or 75 percent of the practicing naturopathic doctors responded affirmatively, whereas the response of the first respondent was evasive, which can make one believe that he may have had no evidence to support such an assertion.

Free radicals destroy cells of DNA with negative repercussions on glands, tissues, and organs. They perform targeted actions on cells of the pancreas, and in the process may damage the pancreas, with diabetes as a result. Toxic particles of the environment such as cadmium, lead and mercury, can cause a chain reaction leading to reformation of free radicals. Other toxins like pesticides, cigarette smoke, alcohol, radiation, and even certain drugs can also lead to free radical accumulation.[73] Absorption of antioxidants like Super ORAC, Super Antioxidant, and N-Acetyl Cysteine may help neutralize free radical damage.

Dehydration may have multiple causes, but foremost is a lack of fluid distribution. Bacteria and viruses may help weaken the digestive system, giving rise to disorders such as Crohn's disease, diverticulitis, etc. in the gastrointestinal tract and decelerate the water absorption capacity of the digestive system.[74] Frequent urination as a result of too much carbohydrate intake may also lead to dehydration. Dehydration can thwart the body biochemical reactions and lead to ailments of any types, such as diabetes. Obtaining a good water filter is a very important decision to make;

---

[73] Diabetes without Drugs: The 5-Step Program to Control Blood Sugar Naturally and Prevent Diabetes Complications—by Suzy Cohen, RPH—2010

[74] A Fighting Chance by Dr. Gordon Pedersen—2008

otherwise it may necessitate the daily intake of chlorophyll to increase the pH level of the water. If bacteria and viruses are present in the digestive system, two teaspoons of Silver Shield with Aqua Sol, in the morning and in the evening, can aid to remedy bacterial and viral infections. Acidophilus, Bifidophilus, and Probiotic Eleven will also help.

Different body parts of the human organism communicate to each other through the nerves (nervous system) and the hormones (hormonal system). But unmanageable stress can affect the nervous system, and the limbic system may become unbalanced due to uncontrollable emotions from the stress.

Hypothesis 7

All respondents agreed that a level of glucose above optimal can result from the concomitant action of ingested foods, dehydration, and the individual's inability to deal with stressful or emotional situations. However, ingested foods and stress-emotions had the most affirmations as factors of diabetes.

Stress and emotion can cause the blood pressure and sugar to go up or down with or without medications or supplements. In some cases, supplements may help relieve such ailments as high blood pressure and high blood sugar. In other cases, Applied Kinesiology[75] has been the only alternative procedure for my colleagues and me.

Deficiencies including stress, emotion, dehydration, and free radicals may act synergistically to cause health problems, such as diabetes. Adequate water consumption and nourishing the nervous system can certainly help in addressing the daily physical and mental health challenges. The companionship of a pet can also help fight the stress and gloom of everyday life. In any case, it is unnecessary to take sleeping pills which are likely to produce hallucinatory and hypnotic effects.

---

[75] Your Body Can Talk—The Art and Application of Clinical Kinesiology—by Susan L. Levy, D. C. and Carl Lehr, M.A.—1996

Summary

All in all, every naturopathic practitioner interviewed agreed with all the hypotheses statements except hypothesis 4. For this hypothesis, the respondents were affirmative with a ratio of 3 to 1; the only respondent who did not explicitly answer 'yes' seemed to affirm when he said that "any damage in one body system can harm another body system." Nevertheless, all these findings each constitute a hypothesis based on clinical results through the interviewed naturopathic doctors. We look forward to further research to confirm them.

CONCLUSIONS

Statistics show diabetes cases are increasing. This study has included multiple predictors as obesity and/or inflammation, heredity, hepatic and glandular conditions, stress-emotion, free radicals, and dehydration. Factors aggravating the damage provoked by aspartame and associated with the massive expansion of the food industry should also be taken into account. Final certainty is unknown whether the above identified factors always act concomitantly or separately. However, the truth about this complex topic—diabetes—involves at least one of these predictors, which can additionally be utilized boldly to establish a basis for subsequent studies on the diabetes phenomena.

Inflammatory chemicals proliferate in food consumption according to some respondents. Monosodium glutamate (MSG), a flavor enhancer in processed foods and canned vegetables, is full of toxic fats. It could be a contributing cause of cell membrane resistance to insulin. This obliges the pancreas to produce more insulin, which may itself become an inflammatory agent as well as the MSG, hydrogenated oils, and inflammatory chemicals impeding food ingestion. Liberating the cell membranes from inflammation may reverse Type II diabetes and allow for a decrease in insulin intake for Type I diabetics. Noni in its liquid form can also help reduce such inflammation.

If obesity or inflammation is the direct result of personal food choices, why do orthodox medicine and the food industry concentrate typically on profit at the cost of public health? The assertion by Dr. Irene Frachon[76] that the mass marketed drug,

---

[76] Dr. Irene Frachon, op. cit.

Mediator, was non effective is a glaring example of the intentional misinformation by the pharmaceutical companies against the public.

Health practitioners should come to realize that the diabetes pandemic cannot be elucidated only through the conclusions of orthodox medicine, which predominantly focused on one being overweight or obese as the main explanations for the diabetes ailment. Most of the swallowed foods are industrial and fortified with preservatives and flavor enhancers making the foods tastier to ensure repeat customers. Rarely does vitamin D appear in this type of diet. Products richest in vitamin D are fatty fish such as cod, salmon or sardines.

Overall, the policies against the pandemic that induces diabetes have failed, including those in the United States. Some interest groups are maneuvering in the shadows and conspiring to sustain the current status. Lobbyists for the food industry encourage personal choice by consumers as this benefits their sponsors.

Prescribing insulin for insulin deficient and non-entirely-insulin deficient diabetics is one of the most common and ongoing mistakes with orthodox medicine. The same way water retention can cause the body to build up more fats than usual to support life, a decrease in blood sugar as a result of insulin intake can cause the body to start secreting growth hormones and a secretion named epinephrine. This secretion maintains the increased blood sugar, which is likely to call for more insulin ingestion and expose diabetic patients to cardiovascular problems, "inner arterial wall damage", and other diabetes related complications affecting the eyes, kidneys and peripheral nerves.[77]

Some drugs have been designed to increase the sensitivity of the so-called receptor sites to allocate more gaps for glucose to enter cells, but instead seem to have created disharmony within cells. In contrast, harmony always comes from a positive mental state. Perfect health is the result of the combined effect of a symbiosis between body, mind and spirit. Healing takes place inside the body

---

[77]   The Complete Encyclopedia of Natural Healing by Gary Null, Ph.D.—2005

and results from the mutual action of body, mind and the spirit. Trying to find a "cure" for cancer or diabetes, for instances, is to engage in a journey with no return.

Dr. Irving Oyle, in his book, entitled "The Healing Man," described the healer—be it a doctor, a physician, a priest, a voodoo priest, a pastor, a naturopath, a shaman, etc.—to be a "channeler" of energy into human bodies. The patient's responsibility is to internalize the healer's actions. The recipient may process it or reject the complete procedure; health has a sacred dimension.

There are different belief systems to promote healing. Examples include medications, exercise, prayer, repeating a mantra, etc or combinations thereof. The will to live is the major reason for healing of any ailments, regardless of the ritual used. The therapist healer is expected to have complete belief in the efficacy of his or her methods. The patient must also have absolute faith in the healer and comprehend the intentions of the latter. The rationale is that faith is the action initiator. If any issue comes up with either person, the healing process may be compromised. From this perspective, healing is not and should never be solely the preserve of physicians.

RECOMMENDATIONS

Generally orthodox medicine recommends that diabetics have a meter reader that allows them to test the level of sugar in their bloodstream at any time. A very high or very low blood sugar or just ten percent rise[78] or fall[79] in the blood glucose is one of the meter characteristics.

Some diabetics test their sugar level several times during a single day, especially early in the morning and at night before bedtime whether or not they take medication or insulin treatment. This process is a counterproductive procedure as it may favor hyperinsulinemia and trigger hypoglycemia.

Diabetics should test the level of glucose in their bloodstream only in the morning upon waking before any meals, to measure the effect of food intake the day before. They should avoid taking medication unless their blood sugar goes beyond 140 mg/dl because the person in question would run out of energy, as a direct effect of insulin intake. But orthodox medicine sees people with a blood sugar between 100-125 mg/dl as pre-diabetics, and considers diabetics to be all those with a blood sugar reaching 126 mg/dl or higher.

Before 1997, a reading beyond 140 milligrams per deciliter of blood defined a diabetic. In 1997 a committee of the World Health

---

[78]   Say over 400 mg/dl
[79]   Say under 50 mg/dl

Organization (WHO) lowered the threshold to 126.[80] Instantly, 1.7 million more American diabetics appeared on the database. Clearly, pharmaceutical companies lower the diagnostic threshold to treat as many patients as possible for as long as possible.

A written diary of their blood sugar readings by diabetics on a healing protocol helps develop patient or client responsibility. Orthodox medicine allows diabetics to eat fruits of any kind, and advises those with Type-I diabetes to test the level of their blood sugar four times a day, and to adjust the amount of insulin based on food intake and physical activity.[81] This is not only counterproductive but also misleading to the entire diabetic population as fruits build up more glucose in the bloodstream and keep diabetics on medications for a lifetime. Therefore diabetics should cut all fruits and commercial juices from their diet, except for papaya, lemons and grapefruits, in order to lower glucose in the bloodstream. Diabetics may take a mixture of the following on any given day between 7:00 a.m. and 11:00 a.m.: celery, carrots, beets, spinach, coconut, and ginger as shown in the supplemental materials provided in this study. As fruits and legumes vary widely in vibration, diabetics should also be aware that some stomach discomfort may arise as a result of ingesting several of them within a short time period.

The diabetic routine should exclude fried foods and starchy foods. Fried foods may alter the total state of the patient by causing blockages in the veins and arteries. Starchy foods may have plenty of starchy substances which are not suitable for diabetics. Among starchy foods are cereal products, spaghetti, cake, nuts, potatoes, sweet potatoes, white yam, yucca, cheese, sweeteners, sugars, peanut butter, white bread, vermicelli, macaroni, mayonnaise,

---

[80] TV5Monde broadcasted on July 7, 2012 in New York a study on the U.S. population. This study led to a confrontation of ideas and responses between journalists and researchers subservient to the orthodox health system. Researchers non-subservient to the orthodox health system were also interviewed, and highlighted the objectives and practices of the drug industry.

[81] The New Glucose Revolution for Diabetes (The Definitive Guide to Managing Diabetes and Pre-diabetes using The Glycemic Index) by Stephen Colagiuri, MD, et al.—2007

banana, plantain, rice, pasta, etc. Diabetics should not consume any starchy foods throughout the period in which they are on a strict personal nutritional regimen determined for their body by Applied Kinesiology. A specific regimen is not always totally appropriate for other diabetics. Applied Kinesiology can help decide on the diabetic's personal tolerance for specific vegetables. The rationale is that Applied Kinesiology has found differences in the glycemic level of some vegetables that seems to vary for many diabetics.

Terminating blood sugar variations in Type-1 diabetes necessitates repairing a damaged chromosome. Concerning gestational diabetes, which may signal stress, pancreatic weakness, and/or iodine deficiency, the thyroid gland and the nervous system should both be well fed. Nutri-Calm and Nervous System are two suitable food supplements for nervous system nourishment, and a long-term combination of Thyroid Activator, or Dulse or Kelp combined with sea salt will be very beneficial to the thyroid gland. Ultimately, only very disciplined people who can strictly follow their *modus operandi* can reverse the diabetes ailment. What is the rationale for this set of recommendations for Type-1 diabetic people?

Unless a newborn has been exposed to toxin and/or heavy metals, such as lead and aluminum, vaccinating a pregnant woman seems to be the only factor that can potentially lead to autoimmune disease. By autoimmune disease, we mean lupus, Crohn's disease, Celiac disease, and Type 1 diabetes. In fact, vaccinating a pregnant woman can damage at least one chromosome; that is, a person's genetic materials. In this case, the pancreas may be unable to produce enough insulin, unless the damaged chromosome or chromosomes have been repaired – which is highly unlikely.

The likelihood of chromosome repair is determined by the ability of the health practitioner to heal or balance the damaged chromosome or chromosomes, and by the willingness of the diabetic person to follow a specific diet, including chromium intake. What is the rationale for chromium intake?

In Type 2 diabetes, however, the pancreas produces enough insulin, but the insulin cannot drive the glucose to the cells to lower the sugar in the blood. Therefore, the sugar accumulates in the blood without any control. Therefore, conventional medicine concludes that the cells, or their receptors, are resisting the insulin, which is wrong because there is no such thing as insulin resistance.

What is really happening in such a scenario is that the body is deficient in chromium. In fact, without chromium, insulin cannot properly drive the glucose into the cell membranes to lower the blood sugar. What do we mean by that?

On average, in case of chromium deficiency, it takes insulin twice as much time to drive glucose into cells. Therefore, it is not the cells or their receptors that are resisting insulin; it is chromium that are deficient in the body. To maintain the blood sugar at a proper level, insulin must be combined with chromium. Such a combination has helped our clients and our former clients experience good health. Nobody can experience good health when chromium is lacking. But most arable land in the United States is deficient in chromium. Similarly, during pregnancy, the fetus may absorb most of the mother's vitamins and minerals' reserve. As a result, the pregnant woman can develop diabetic like symptoms, hypertension like symptoms and even eclampsia, which is seizure like symptoms that looks like epilepsy. Pregnant women who are diagnosed with mineral deficiency also known as anemia are likely to develop eclampsia at the time of giving birth. All in all, anemia can by itself trigger diabetes. Chromium deficiency can by itself trigger diabetes. Anemia, chromium, and zinc deficiency can concomitantly further alter the apparent ability of insulin to drive glucose into the cell membranes. Note that drugstore chromium and zinc can be detrimental to human health.

Diabetics ought to make choices that display personal maturation. In other words, the healing protocol should be used as a guideline for entering a new lifestyle. Avoidance of foods outside of their healing protocol that can add weight is an exercise of their will to stay with their new diet, as any deviation might be prejudicial. In fact, although not all of my diabetic clients have rigorously followed any proposed healing protocol, most of them are happy with just feeling better.

Any diabetic who wants to get over this ailment needs to stick 100 percent to the healing protocol assigned to them. The rationale for this is that such a protocol is personal, and is established for that particular diabetic through Applied Kinesiology. In other words, as the assigned protocol is personal, it cannot be arbitrarily used to help heal another diabetic since the glycemic level of various foods varies from one diabetic to another.

Diabetics who neglect to abide by the recommendations indicated above may see their blood glucose remain high for a long duration, or vary within a range that may still exceed its ideal level. Perhaps in either case, the sensitive nerves may be altered to the point that they no longer send out pain signals and give warnings for cold or hot body conditions. Sores may develop, perhaps leading to the so-called gangrene usually associated with the last stage before amputation.

The strict implementation of the stated recommendations would have a redundancy on most diseases known to man. Furthermore, it will indubitably allow blood to flow to the entire body in order to conceivably prevent the complications that too often are related to diabetes: numbness, heart attack, gangrene, leg ulcers, kidney malfunction, congestive heart failure, neurologic dysfunction, blind spots or loss of sight, and improper coordination of movement.

INDEX

A

acid reflux, 19

ancestors, 10, 84

anemia, 74

angina, 43

applied kinesiology, 5, 6, 36, 43, 52, 66, 72, 73,

aspartame, 26, 27, 32, 33, 34, 35, 44, 68

atrophic gastritis, 21

B

bacteria, 11, 20, 21, 28, 39, 60, 64, 65

benfluorex, 24, 25

beta cells, 6, 37, 38, 39

bifidobacteria, 39

blind spots, 74

blood glucose, 7, 27, 37, 41, 42, 56, 57, 60, 62, 71, 74

blood sugar, 6, 10, 11, 12, 24, 26, 27, 36, 37, 38, 39, 41, 42, 53, 55, 57, 58, 59, 61, 66, 69, 71, 72, 73

Body Mass Index (BMI), 12

C

carbohydrates, 9, 16, 26, 34, 35, 36, 52, 56, 60

chromium, 74

chromosome, 73

constipation, 22, 28, 30

contingent factor, 8, 46, 47, 50

D

dehydration, 8, 11, 28, 46, 48, 53, 56, 59, 64, 65, 66, 68

descendants, 10, 48, 54

diabetes, 6, 7, 8, 9, 10, 12, 13, 15, 18, 24, 26, 27, 28, 30, 34, 36, 37, 38, 40, 41, 42, 43, 46, 47, 50, 52, 53, 54, 55, 56, 57, 59, 61, 63, 64, 66, 68, 69, 70, 72, 73, 74

digestion, 19, 20, 21, 22, 23, 30, 33, 61

diverticulitis, 19, 65

drugs, 19, 20, 21, 23, 24, 25, 26, 28, 29, 32, 41, 44, 45, 65, 70

E

eclampsia, 74

emotions, 8, 11, 53, 65, 66

endocrine glands, 10, 61

enzymes, 19, 20, 21, 22, 28, 30, 39, 42, 44, 59, 60, 63

erectile dysfunction, 19

excess glucose, 42, 55

T

type 1 diabetes, 30, 73
type 2 diabetes, 31, 74
toxic chemicals, 22
toxins, 19, 21, 35, 39, 60, 65
trans-fats, 23, 29

V

vitamins, 5, 10, 12, 18, 23, 29, 33
vitamin C, 17, 30, 31, 44
vitamin E, 43, 44

BIBLIOGRAPHY

1. Completing Your Doctoral Dissertation or Master's Thesis in two semesters or less by Dr. Evelyn Hunt Ogden, 1993—Second Edition

2. L'enquête en psycho-sociologie by Hélène Chauchat—Presse Universitaire de France, 1985

3. An Introduction to Statistics by Mason, Lind, and Marchal, 1983

4. Encyclopedia of Natural Medicine by Murray and Pizzorno, 1991

5. Diabetes Solution: The Complete Guide to Archiving Normal Blood Sugar by Richard K. Bernstein, MD, 2007

6. Diabetes Without Drugs: The 5—Step Program to Control Blood Sugar Naturally and Prevent Diabetes Complications by Suzy Cohen, 2010

7. The John Hopkins Guide to Diabetes For Today and Tomorrow by Christopher D. Sandek, M. D., Richard R. Rubin, Ph. D., CDE, Cynthia S. Shump, R.N., CDE, and Johns Hopkins Press Health Book, 1997

8. The Everything Guide to Managing and Reversing Pre-Diabetes by Gretchen Scalpi, RD, CDN, CDE, 2011

9. Toxic by WILLIAM REYMOND, 2010

10. Essential Endocrinology and Diabetes (Essentials) by Richard I.G. Holt, 2007

11. The Complete Diabetes Prevention Plan: A Guide to Understanding the Emerging Epidemic of Pre-diabetes and Halting Its Pr by Sandra Woodruff, Christopher Saudek, 2005

12. The New Glucose Revolution Pocket Guide to the Metabolic Syndrome by Ph.D. Jennie Brand-Miller Ph.D., Kaye Foster-Powell M. Nutrition & Diet, Anthony Leeds, Kaye Foster-Powell B.SC. M. Nutri. & Diet, 2011

13. Cooking for Diabetics (Food & drink) by Kitty Maynard, Lucian Maynard, Theodore G. Duncan, Julia M. Pitkin, 2011

14. Losing Weight with Your Diabetes Medication: How Byetta and Other Drugs Can Help You Lose More Weight than You Ever Thought Possible (Marlowe Diabetes Library) by David Mendosa, M.D. Joe Prendergast, 2011

15. Diabetes Mellitus: A Practical Handbook by Sue K. Milchovich RN BSN CDE, Barbara Dunn-Long RD, 2011

16. Oxford Handbook of Endocrinology and Diabetes (Oxford Handbooks) by Helen Turner, John Wass, 2011

17. Insulin Resistance: the Metabolic Syndrome X (Contemporary Endocrinology) by Gerald M. Reaven, Ami Laws, 2011

18. Diabetes Management: Clinical Pathways, Guidelines, and Patient Education (Aspen Chronic Disease Management Series) by Health and Administration Development Group (Aspen Publishers), Jo Gulledge, Shawn Beard, 2011

19. Action Plan for Diabetes (Action Plan for Health Series) by Darryl Barnes, 2011

20. A Study of Metabolism in Severe Diabetes by Francis Gano Benedict, 2011

21. Living Well With Diabetes: A Practical Guide For Physical And Spiritual Renewal by Rosalia J. Coffen, 2011

22. Clinical Diabetes Research: Methods and Techniques by Michael Roden, 2011

23. Diabetes: The New Type 2: Your Complete Handbook to Living Healthfully with Diabetes Type 2 by Virginia Valentine, June Biermann, Barbara Toohey, 2011

24. Type 1 Diabetes, An Issue of Endocrinology Clinics by Desmond A. Schatz, Michael Haller, and Mark Atkinson, 2011

25. Type 1 Diabetes, An Issue of Endocrinology Clinics by Desmond A. Schatz, Michael Haller, and Mark Atkinson, 2011

26. Dr. Neal Barnard's Program for Reversing Diabetes by Neal D. Banard, M. D., 2007

27. The Healing Power of Exercise: Your Guide to Preventing and Treating Diabetes, Depression, Heart Disease, High Blood Pressure, and More by Linn Goldberg, Diane L. Elliot, 2011

28. The Healing Power of Exercise, 2011

29. Combining Old and New: Naturopathy in the 21st Century, by Robert J. Thiel, PhD, 2011

30. Putting It All Together, by Hoffer & Walker, 2011

31. Advanced Treatise in Herbology, by Dr. Edward Shook, 2011

32. Your Health, Your Choice, by Dr. Ted Morter, 2011

33. Prescription for Nutritional Healing (4th edition), by James and Phyllis Balch, 2011

34. A Cancer Battle Plan, by Anne and David Frahm, 2011

35. Science and Practice of Iridology, by Dr. Bernard Jensen, 2011

36. Nutritional Herbology, by Mark Pedersen, ND, 2011

37. Homeopathic Medicine at Home, by Dr. Maesimund Panos and Jane Heimlich, 2011

38. Nutrition in Action, by Kurt W. Donsbach, DC, ND, PhD, 2011

39. The Complete Encyclopedia of Natural Healing, by Gary Null, PhD, 2005

40. Ultimate Healing System, by Dr. Donald Lepore, 2011

41. Dry Blood Cell Analysis, by CRNH, 2004 Edition

42. Herbal Medicine Maker's Handbook, by James Green, 2011

43. Enzymes the Key to Health, by Howard F. Loomis, Jr. DC, FIACA, 2011

44. Chemistry of Man, by Bernard Jensen, Copyright 2007

45. Advanced Bach Flower Therapy, by Gotz Blome, M.D.

46. The Healing Mind, by Dr. Irving Oyle

47. Diet and Nutrition, by Dr. Rudolph Ballentine, 2010

48. Planetary Herbology, by Michael Tierra,1992

49. The New Bible Cure for Diabetes by Don Colbert M.D., 1982, by Thomas Nelson, Inc.

50. The New Glucose Revolution for Diabetes by Dr. Jennie Brand-Miller, PhD Kaye Foster-Powell, M. Nutri & Diet Stephen Colagiuri, M.D., Alan W. Barclay, Bsci, Grad Dip Diabetics, 2007

51. Understanding Diabetes by Marie Clark, 2004

52. The End of Overeating: Taking Control of the Insatiable American Appetite by David A. Kessler, 2010

APPENDIX

APPENDIX 1

INTERVIEW GRID

1. What factors may cause Type II diabetes, besides food consumption and obesity?

2. How can obesity cause pancreatic damage?

3. How does the type I diabetes differ from type 2 diabetes?

4. How does gestational diabetes mellitus differ from the other types, and what kinds of people are likely to develop this type of diabetes?

5. When can someone be considered pre-diabetic, and why?

6. Which known conditions might lead to diabetes?

7. Which environmental factors are likely to elevate the blood sugar levels and eventually lead to diabetes?

8. We know that pathogens like bacteria, viruses, fungi, and parasites attempt to invade our bodies to disrupt homeostasis and cause disease. Other pathogens release toxins (poisons) in the body. Some other pathogens trigger fevers. Can internal factors such as pathogens play a role in diabetes development?

9. We know that free radicals can destroy the DNA within the cell. Can the pancreas become diseased as a result?

10. Can heavy metals such as cadmium, lead, and mercury cause pancreatic damage as well? Why or why not?

11. A medical doctor named Dr. Mercola reported based on research results that statin drugs raise blood sugar, while the pancreas may be working properly. Have you experienced the same thing in your practice?

12. Many people are mineral deficient. Some of them are so deficient that their heart is affected. Since mineral deficiency is a systemic problem, can it result in diabetes? Why or why not?

13. Iodine deficiency negatively affects the thyroid gland, which signals the heart for proper blood circulation and oxygen and nutrient transport. Can a weak thyroid indirectly add to pancreatic damage? Why or why not?

14. Usually the liver cleans toxins out of the body. A damaged liver possibly contributes to high cholesterol and toxin build up. Is a damaged liver an open door for pancreatic damage? Why or why not?

15. Some diabetics are insulin-resistant. How does this resistance to insulin absorption come into play?

16. It seems that many people diagnosed with diabetes progress through life blindly. They do not know what to do. We heard someone say that his sugar level increases whether he eats or not. What do you recommend for the daily life of a diabetic?

17. For you, what is the leading cause (s) of diabetes? Question 17 will serve as a brief review or summary.

18. How many people did you help with this modality, Applied Kinesiology? Choose one

    Respondent #1: __Hardly helped at all __Helped to some extent __Helped to a great extent

    Respondent #2: __Hardly helped at all __Helped to some extent __Helped to a great extent

    Respondent #3: __Hardly helped at all __Helped to some extent __Helped to a great extent

    Respondent #4: __Hardly helped at all __Helped to some extent __Helped to a great extent

19. What percent of your clients got better?

Respondent #1:
__Less than 10% __Between 10 and 20% __Between 20 and 30%
__About 50% __More than 50% __Between 65 and 75%
__Between 75 and 85% __Between 85 and 95% __100%

Respondent #2:
__Less than 10% __Between 10 and 20% __Between 20 and 30%
__About 50% __More than 50% __Between 65 and 75%
__Between 75 and 85% __Between 85 and 95% __100%

Respondent #3:
__Less than 10% __Between 10 and 20% __Between 20 and 30%
__About 50% __More than 50% __Between 65 and 75% *
__Between 75 and 85% __Between 85 and 95% __100%

Respondent #4:
__Less than 10% __Between 10 and 20% __Between 20 and 30%
__About 50% __More than 50% __Between 65 and 75%
__Between 75 and 85% __Between 85 and 95% __100%

20. What improvement(s) justified your choice in question #19? Choose all that apply

Respondent #1:
__Clients changed their diet as a result
__They no longer have to take insulin, but food supplements
__They no longer on medications for diabetes
__Cells assimilate insulin produced
__Proper diet helps them to maintain their blood sugar at normal level
__They lost weight
__Their pancreas produced enough insulin

Respondent #2:

__Clients changed their diet as a result

__They no longer have to take insulin, but food supplements

__They no longer on medications for diabetes

__Cells assimilate insulin produced

__Proper diet helps them to maintain their blood sugar at normal level

__They lost weight

__Their pancreas produced enough insulin

Respondent #3:

__Clients changed their diet as a result

__They no longer have to take insulin, but food supplements

__They no longer on medications for diabetes

__Cells assimilate insulin produced

__Proper diet helps them to maintain their blood sugar at normal level

__They lost weight

__Their pancreas produced enough insulin

Respondent #4:

__Clients changed their diet as a result

__They no longer have to take insulin, but food supplements

__They no longer on medications for diabetes

__Cells assimilate insulin produced

__Proper diet helps them to maintain their blood sugar at normal level

__They lost weight

__Their pancreas produced enough insulin

APPENDIX 2

INTERVIEW TRANSCRIPT VERBATIM

Responses to open-ended questions asked during the interview series from my recording device make up the corpus with which I worked to test the hypotheses.

I arranged the following data by Units of Analysis.

1. What factors may cause type II diabetes, besides food consumption and obesity?

Respondent #1: Stress, emotion, worries, spleen, liver, any accident affecting the ribs, a shock (emotional or physical), gallbladder, kidney, adrenal glands, thyroid, medications, dehydration, bacteria, fungi, parasites, lack of minerals, lack of vitamins, presence of free radicals in the body, and body structure may be involved in Type 2 diabetes. To justify his long response, Respondent #1 said, "The body is like an orchestra, where several musicians are playing a partition. If one of them plays the partition wrong, the whole partition 'falls.' "In this statement, the doctor implied that diabetes could be caused by any abnormal body function."

Respondent #2: Only adults happen to have Type 2 diabetes. The pancreas may produce insulin, and the insulin produced is not effective, which may cause sugar to accumulate in the bloodstream perhaps because of lack fluid (dehydration) or fluid distribution to enhance transport. In addition, injustices suffered by our ancestors can cause problems particularly in both the reproductive and digestive systems of their descendants. Consider a woman who may have lived in slavery at one time and possibly raped by her master (historical factors). This woman may have suffered an emotional shock that was transmitted from generation to generation (heredity). Medications are possibly another cause of diabetes.

Respondent #3: Many things can cause type II diabetes; emotion is one of them; obesity is another. Socio-economic problems, associated with historical factors that generate emotional stress and frustrations, can also cause diabetes.

Respondent #4: Only adults develop type II diabetes. Type II diabetes is therefore called adult onset diabetes. Emotional discomfort may be a historical factor of diabetes development, but malnutrition causes about 80 percent of obesity, which leads to type II diabetes. Junk foods and dehydration can contribute to indigestion, which means diabetes is a digestive disease. The blood stream of diabetics may be unable to digest sugar and fats due to a weak liver or an imbalance in the pancreas itself.

2. How can obesity cause pancreatic damage?

    Respondent #1: The pancreas produces little or no insulin at all.

    Respondent #2: The pancreas is under pressure to produce more and more insulin.

    Respondent #3: Excess carbohydrates promote weight gain, which triggers obesity that damages the pancreas.

    Respondent #4: The blood stream of diabetics is unable to digest sugar and fats.

3. How does the type I diabetes differ from type 2 diabetes?

    Respondent #1: For type I diabetes, the body has been unable to recognize and absorb chromium at birth (heredity), but the pancreas cannot function without it. Only children can develop type 1 or juvenile diabetes. The medical profession considers children experiencing this ailment as insulin dependent. However, some adults with type 2 diabetes have become insulin dependent as well because of stress and emotion that affect the pancreas. Another reason could be that they have too many simple carbohydrates in their diet, which cause the pancreas to stop producing insulin, leading to the rise in blood sugar past the ideal level. Since the blood sugar remains high, these type 2 people are on insulin as well, and are also called insulin dependent; they wrongly refer to those adult diabetics as being type 1.

Respondent #2: For type 1 diabetes, the body does not recognize chromium because of a damaged chromosome (heredity). And type 2 is mostly caused by bad diet, which triggers the obesity that affects the pancreas.

Respondent #3: Type 1, to the contrary of type 2, is the result of a damaged chromosome at birth (heredity). Only children can develop it. From this we get the name, juvenile diabetes.

Damaged Islets of Langerhans, groups of specialized cells in the pancreas cause type I diabetes because the pancreas has never been able to produce insulin since birth or at an early age.

Respondent #4: Type I diabetes is genetic; only children are likely to develop this type of diabetes. Another name for Type 1 is juvenile diabetes. The hereditary nature of type I diabetes affects the children's chromosomes. Damaged Islets of Langerhans, specialized groups of cells in the pancreas cause type I diabetes because the pancreas has never been able to produce insulin since birth or at an early age. Orthodox medicine believes these children usually stay on insulin for life. However, proper food ingestion, food supplements, supported by Applied Kinesiology can help to reverse type I diabetes.

4. How does the gestational diabetes mellitus differ from the other types, and what kinds of individuals are most likely to develop this type of diabetes?

Respondent #1: Only pregnant women so far have developed gestational diabetes; such difficulty occurs during pregnancy and is due to a thyroid weakness.

Respondent #2: The thyroid gland causes diabetes and mostly during pregnancy. Thyroid dysfunction may affect the entire body, especially the pancreas, during pregnancy. So, in case of gestational diabetes, one needs to pay attention to the thyroid while supporting the pancreas with Blood Sugar Formula, Pro Pancreas, and Chromium.

Respondent #3: Gestational diabetes only afflicts pregnant women. The thyroid gland is responsible for it.

Respondent #4: Only pregnant women are likely to develop gestational diabetes. Three months after pregnancy, an embryo becomes a fetus. From this point on until birth, the formation of tissues and organs is dependent on the mother's nutritional intake. Therefore, pregnant women must make proper nutrition high on their list of priorities. Women who developed diabetes before pregnancy already had a weakness in the pancreas; they may be chromium deficient. Before they get pregnant, women must make sure that their body has everything it needs in terms of nutrition to feed the fetus. Among those women diagnosed with gestational diabetes, some remain diabetics; others sometimes recover after having gestational diabetes, but are still likely to develop type II diabetes anytime afterwards.

5. When can someone be considered pre-diabetic, and why?

Respondent #1: The blood sugar is high because the pancreas did not produce enough insulin or the insulin that is produced has not been distributed properly.

Respondent #2: Obesity or emotional stress has caused the blood sugar to go high

Respondent #3: Pre-diabetes often indicates a sedentary life, lack of exercise, poor eating habits, and too much carbohydrate intake.

Respondent #4: Pre-diabetics have their blood sugar 'between' 100-125. This depends on the time of day the test occurs. The glucose level of all 'healthy' people can go beyond 110 or 115 depending on consumption. In other words, the pancreas may produce excess insulin in a normal person to adapt to an overflow of glucose. Then the pancreas produces insulin and an enzyme called amylase to balance any excess insulin in the blood and prevents diabetes development. Otherwise a pre-diabetic condition may occur.

6. Which known conditions might lead to diabetes?

Respondent #1: Worries, stress, emotions, dehydration, shock and trauma; anything can cause anything

Respondent #2: Failure to drink plenty of water, anxieties, being overweight, and medications

Respondent #3: Repressed desires for emancipation/ sedentary life/ metabolic problems/ poor eating habits

Respondent #4: Poor diet, a fatty liver, weight gain, malnutrition can all lead to diabetes.

7. Which environmental factors are likely to elevate the blood sugar levels and eventually lead to diabetes?

    Respondent #1: Ionizing radiation in the environment, in the water we drink, in the sun, in the food we eat, in addition to free radicals and toxic particles

    Respondent #2: Free radicals, radiation, and toxic wastes can lead to blood sugar elevation

    Respondent #3: Free radicals, ionizing radiations are environmental contributors to diabetes, and are known to elevate the blood sugar levels.

    Respondent #4; Viruses and bacteria in the environment can attack the pancreas or any other organs and cause diabetes. Likewise, excessive time exposed to smoke, free radicals in the environment, and toxins in our drinking water may also make one become diabetic.

8. We know that pathogens like bacteria, viruses, fungi, and parasites attempt to invade our bodies to disrupt homeostasis and cause disease. Other pathogens release toxins (poisons) in the body. Some other pathogens trigger fevers. Can internal factors such as pathogens play a role in diabetes development?

    Respondent #1: I already said it: anything can cause anything.

    Respondent #2: Definitely

    Respondent #3: Blockages due to parasites, fungi, or viruses may cause the Islets of Langerhans to not work properly.

    Respondent #4: Viruses and bacteria in the environment can attack the pancreas or any other organs and cause diabetes.

9. We know that free radicals can destroy the DNA within the cell. Can the pancreas become diseased as a result?

   <u>Respondent #1</u>: Quite possible, anything can cause anything.

   <u>Respondent #2</u>: It is clearly stated in literature on diabetes that free radicals can destroy the DNA within the cell and cause damages anywhere in the digestive system

   <u>Respondent #3</u>: Obviously, yes!

   <u>Respondent #4</u>: Free radicals in the environment and toxins in our drinking water may as well become diabetic factors.

10. Can heavy metals such as cadmium, lead, and mercury cause pancreatic damage as well? Why or why not?

    <u>Respondent #1</u>: Foreign invaders can undermine metabolism and cause diseases, such as diabetes

    <u>Respondent #2</u>: We know that cadmium can damage the kidneys, and a damaged DNA can undermine metabolic procedures and cause dysfunctions anywhere in the body, such as the pancreas

    <u>Respondent #3</u>: I have never checked for those things specifically, but it is quite possible.

    <u>Respondent #4</u>: Smoke exposure, free radicals in the environment, and toxins in our drinking water may as well lead to diabetes.

11. A medical doctor named Dr. Mercola reported based on research results that statin drugs raise blood sugar, while the pancreas may be working properly. Have you experienced the same thing in your practice?

    <u>Respondent #1</u>: Statin drugs are known to cause several turbulences in the body, especially blood sugar elevation.

    <u>Respondent #2</u>: Respondent #2: Statin drugs can help to lower cholesterol, but in the process can damage the liver and cause blood sugar elevation, even while the pancreas may be properly working.

<u>Respondent #3</u>: Medications are disruptive to the entire body.

<u>Respondent #4</u>: About 80 percent of our cholesterol is produced by the liver. Taking statin drugs to reduce cholesterol can affect the functioning of the liver and lead to diabetes.

12. Many people are mineral deficient. Some of them are so deficient that their heart is affected. Since mineral deficiency is a systemic problem, can it result in diabetes? Why or why not?

<u>Respondent #1</u>: Absolutely, because any organs can be affected by mineral and vitamin deficiencies

<u>Respondent #2</u>: It is true that mineral deficiency can negatively affect metabolism and cause weaknesses in organs

<u>Respondent #3</u>: Lack of minerals causes general weakness in the body, which can lead to diabetes.

<u>Respondent #4</u>: Chromium is a mineral of choice for the pancreas. Therefore, any deficiency in the chromium can cause diabetes. Cropland in the United States is deficient in chromium.

13. Iodine deficiency negatively affects the thyroid gland, which signals the heart for proper blood circulation and oxygen and nutrient transport. Can a weak thyroid indirectly add to pancreatic damage? Why or why not?

<u>Respondent #1</u>: Not only can a weak thyroid cause diabetes, the entire glandular system can cause it.

<u>Respondent #2</u>: Most people are living with a weak thyroid without knowing it. Thyroid controls the entire reproductive system. All body systems interact with each other, so any damage in one system may cause harm in another system

<u>Respondent #3</u>: Not just the thyroid. The entire glandular system can cause pancreatic damage. The adrenal glands help remove glucose from the bloodstream, so they can cause diabetes when not working or when not working properly.

<u>Respondent #4</u>: Hypothyroidism slows down the functioning of all organs of the body. So a slowdown in the liver can cause fat accumulation in this organ, and increase the

level of cholesterol but slow down the production and/ or distribution of insulin in the blood. Excessive exposure to stressful and/or emotional situations, such as loss of a loved one or the inability to cope with certain aspects of life, causes the adrenal glands to produce two of the most powerful hormones, cortisone and adrenalin. The adrenal gland triggers everything in your body to work faster: the heart will work faster, and the liver, which has 600 to 700 different functions, is then stimulated to produce more cholesterol, and the person may experience an increase in the blood pressure. That is why some people develop high cholesterol without eating junk food. This is how secondary factors may lead to diabetes.

14. Usually the liver cleans toxins out of the body. A damaged liver possibly contributes to high cholesterol and toxin build up. Is a damaged liver an open door for pancreatic damage? Why or why not?

Respondent #1: The liver is part of the digestive system. Anything that goes wrong with any parts of the digestive system can directly or indirectly affect the pancreas. When the pancreas doesn't produce at all, it affects the entire digestive system including the liver.

Respondent #2: Both the liver and the pancreas are in the digestive system. Problems in one can negatively harm the other.

Respondent #3: The liver may play a role in diabetes, mostly when it fails to properly remove toxins.

Respondent #4: Obesity causes the liver to become fatty, which causes the receptors in the liver to no longer be able to receive messages from the pancreas properly. The liver is usually able to interact with the pancreas, and is not supposed to paralyze the actions of the pancreas. Obesity however causes more damages to the liver than to the pancreas.

15. Some diabetics are insulin-resistant. How does this resistance to insulin absorption come into play?

Respondent #1: Either there is insufficient insulin production to drive excess glucose into the cells or the cells are just resistant to insulin.

Respondent #2: Cells resist absorbing insulin.

Respondent #3: Insulin resistance is a body reaction that shows that the cause of the diabetes ailment has not been addressed.

Respondent #4: Obesity causes resistance to insulin. Insulin is a foreign body which tends to stop the pancreas' function to produce insulin Therefore it is normal that the body takes time to adapt to this foreign body that it itself did not produce. The body can become resistant to insulin for a while, or for a long time depending on whether the dosage used has been too high and whether the assimilation capacity of our cells decreases.

16. It seems that many people diagnosed with diabetes progress through life blindly; they simply do not know what to do. I recently heard someone say that his sugar level increases whether he eats or not. What do you recommend for the daily life of a diabetic?

Respondent #1: No ingestion of simple carbohydrates during the entire protocol of treatment

Respondent #2: Avoid eating simple carbohydrates, and eat more vegetables

Respondent #3: Eat less and less simple carbohydrates, and increase water intake

Respondent #4; No commercial juice, mix beets with a lot of raw vegetables, fruit juices without sugar to drink in the morning before 1:00 pm, and do not eat at night before going to bed.

17. For you, what are the leading causes of diabetes? Question 17 will serve as a brief review or summary.

Respondent #1: The brain does little or no synchronization of ingested foods

Respondent #2: Obesity, stress and emotions, medications

Respondent #3: Emotions and stress: the pancreas is a sweet organ. Chromium helps to relax it. So lack of sweetness, stress, anxieties, and emotions that go deep into the pancreas can each lead to pancreas malfunction.

Respondent #4: Malnutrition is the number one factor of diabetes.

18. How many people did you help with this modality, Applied Kinesiology? Choose one

Respondent #1:
__Hardly helped at all __Helped to some extent __Helped to a great extent ( )

Respondent #2:
__Hardly helped at all __Helped to some extent __Helped to a great extent ( )

Respondent #3:
__Hardly helped at all __Helped to some extent ( ) __ Helped to a great extent

Respondent #4:
__Hardly helped at all __Helped to some extent ( ) __ Helped to a great extent

19. What percent of your clients got better?

Respondent #1:
__Less than 10% __Between 10 and 20% __Between 20 and 30%
__About 50% __More than 50% __Between 65 and 75%
__Between 75 and 85% __Between 85 and 95% __100%

Respondent #2:
__Less than 10% __Between 10 and 20% __Between 20 and 30%
__About 50% __More than 50% __Between 65 and 75%
__Between 75 and 85% __Between 85 and 95% __100%

Respondent #3:

__Less than 10% __Between 10 and 20% __Between 20 and 30%

__About 50% __More than 50% __Between 65 and 75% *

__Between 75 and 85% __Between 85 and 95% __100%

Respondent #4:

__Less than 10% __Between 10 and 20% __Between 20 and 30%

__About 50% __More than 50% __Between 65 and 75%

__Between 75 and 85% __Between 85 and 95% __100%

20. What improvement(s) justified your choice in question #19? Choose all that apply

Respondent #1:

✓ __Clients changed their diet as a result

✓ __They no longer have to take insulin, but food supplements

✓ __They are no longer on medications for diabetes

✓ __Cells assimilate the insulin produced

✓ __Proper diet helps them to maintain their blood sugar at normal levels

✓ __They lost weight

✓ __Their pancreas produced enough insulin

Respondent #2:

✓ __Clients changed their diet as a result

✓ __They no longer have to take insulin, but food supplements

✓ __They are no longer on medications for diabetes

✓ __Cells assimilate the insulin produced

✓ __Proper diet helps them to maintain their blood sugar at normal levels

✓ __They lost weight

✓ __Their pancreas produced enough insulin

Respondent #3:

✓ __Clients changed their diet as a result

✓ __They no longer have to take insulin, but food supplements

✓ __They no longer on medications for diabetes

✓ __Cells assimilate the insulin produced
✓ __Proper diet helps them to maintain their blood sugar at normal levels
✓ __They lost weight
✓ __Their pancreas produced enough insulin

Respondent #4:
✓ __Clients changed their diet as a result
✓ __They no longer have to take insulin, but food supplements
✓ __They no longer on medications for diabetes
✓ __Cells assimilate the insulin produced
✓ __Proper diet helps them to maintain their blood sugar at normal levels
✓ __They lost weight
✓ __Their pancreas produced enough insulin

APPENDIX 3

CATEGORIES

The following is a set of coded information from the interview transcripts constructed into ten written categories; the size of each is dependent on the data collection format. The adjusted categories break off the overlapping information in the interview transcripts.

1. Categories for factors involved in type II diabetes
   - Food consumption and obesity
   - Stress and emotion
   - Dehydration
   - Adrenal imbalance
   - Vitamins and mineral deficiencies
   - Bacteria and or parasites
   - Toxins and free radicals
   - Body misalignment
   - Medications
   - Other (describe) _____

   Check all that apply.

2. Categories for pancreatic damaged
   - Food consumption and obesity
   - Too little insulin produced
   - No insulin is produced
   - Heavy metals (such as cadmium, lead, and mercury, etc.)
   - Destructive actions of free radicals (to the DNA within the cell)
   - Liver damaged
   - Other (describe) _____

   Check all that apply.

3. Categories for differentiation between type I and type II diabetes

Type I Diabetes	Type II Diabetes
—The body no longer recognized chromium —Other (describe) _____	Same categories as for question 1

Check all that apply.

4. Categories for differentiation between the gestational diabetes mellitus and the other types of diabetes

Gestational Diabetes Mellitus	Type I Diabetes	Type II Diabetes
—Pregnant Women —Thyroid Weakness —Other (describe) _____	Same categories as for question 3	Same categories as for question 1

Check all that apply.

5. Categories for determining pre-diabetic
   - Not enough insulin produced
   - Improper distribution of insulin
   - Blood sugar elevation between 100 and 125 mg/dl
   - Other (describe) _____

Check all that apply.

6. Categories for environmental factors
   - Heavy metals (such as cadmium, lead, and mercury)
   - Toxic particles and free radicals

- Bacteria and viruses
- Other (describe) _____

Check all that apply

7. Categories for internal factors such as pathogens
   - Toxins from bacteria and the cells
   - Bacteria, fungi, viruses, and parasites (disrupt homeostasis)
   - Other (describe)

Check all that apply.

8. Categories for insulin-resistance
   - Not enough insulin produced
     (to drive excess glucose into cells)
   - The cells are resistant to insulin
   - Defecations from bacteria and or parasites block the Islets
     of Langerhans
   - Other (describe) _____

Check all that apply.

9. Categories for daily life of a diabetic person
   - No ingestion of simple carbohydrates
     (during the entire protocol of treatment)
   - No ingestion of fruits at all
   - No ingestion of fruits, except grapefruit and lemon
   - No ingestion of fruits after 1:00p.m. (to allow enough
     time for the body to metabolize excess glucose)
   - Other (describe) _____

Check all that apply.

10. Categories for the leading cause of diabetes
    - Food consumption
    - Obesity
    - Pathogens
    - Vitamin deficiency

- Mineral deficiency
- Adrenal imbalance
- Liver imbalance
- Environmental factors
- Medications
- Worry
- Body structure
- Other (describe) _____

Check only one.

The analyzed interview transcripts highlight the presence and the frequency of specific terms or concepts. Frequency is counting the number of occurrences of an event. Terms or words with the highest frequency are color-coded, definite or indefinite articles are excluded, and synonyms are determined as follows.

I categorized the responses: junk foods, food consumption, malnutrition, weight, obesity, poor diet and poor eating habits as synonymous. The words stress and emotions fell into another group. Therefore, they were grouped as having the same characteristics. The answers: too little insulin, no insulin production or excess productions of it, all have similar impact on the pancreas. Therefore, they fall together in the same class. Pathogens are classified by the words: bacteria, fungi, viruses, and parasites.

To analyze and interpret the characteristics of units, I broke each down into pertinent segments to test the hypotheses. I used numbers to find how many respondents per unit made that choice. For example, Type II Diabetes is a unit by itself and Pancreatic Damages is another.

I based percentages and comparisons on the number of word or phrase occurrences to determine the direction and intensity of these words or phrases. I used frequency and percentages of words or phrases for comparison.

APPENDIX 4

SIMILARITIES AND DIFFERENCES: WORDS AND PHRASES

Similarities	Differences
Type II Diabetes	
Obesity (2), Malnutrition (2), Dehydration (2) Stress-Emotions (2)	Spleen, Liver, Kidneys, Adrenal Glands, Thyroid, Medications, Bacteria, Fungi, Parasites, Lack of Minerals, Free Radicals, Misalignment, Ineffectiveness of Insulin, Dehydration, Improper fluid distribution, Historical factors, Frustrations, Indigestion
Pancreatic Damages	
Insulin Production (3)	Indigestion
Type I Diabetes	
Chromium Assimilation (2), Damaged Chromosomes (2)	Lack of Chromium absorption, Hereditary, Islets of Langerhans are damaged
Gestational Diabetes	
Thyroid Weakness (3)	Pancreatic weakness, Chromium Deficiency
Pre-Diabetic	
Obesity (2)	Not enough insulin produced, Improper Distribution of Insulin, Stress-Emotions, Sedentary Life, Lack of Exercise, Overflow of Glucose
Main Causes of Diabetes	

Weight Gain (4), Dehydration (2)	Stress-Emotions, Medications, Repressed Desire for Emancipation, Sedentary Life, Metabolic Problems, A Fatty Liver
Environmental Factors	
Free radicals (3), (Ionizing) Radiations (2) Toxic Particles (2)	Bacteria, Viruses, Toxins, Smoke Exposure
Internal Factors or Pathogens	
Pathogens (4)	
Free Radicals	
Obviously, yes (2)	Quite Possible, It is a Possibility
Heavy Metals	
Undermine Metabolic Procedures (2)	Never Checked for Those Things, Damage the Pancreas
Medications	
Liver Dysfunction (2)	Blood Sugar Elevation, Disruptions in the Entire Body
Mineral or Vitamin Deficiencies	
General Weakness to the Body (2)	Chromium Deficiency, Affect Organs
A Weak Thyroid	
Affect Glandular System (2), Slows Down Organ Functions (2)	Controls Entire Reproductive System
Liver Damaged	
Pancreatic damage (3)	Accumulate Toxins

Insulin: Resistance	
Cell Resistance (2) Inappropriate Treatment (2)	Under production of insulin
The Daily Life of Diabetic Patients	
No Fruits, Except two of them (2), Vegetables (2) No Commercial Juice (2)	No Ingestion of Simple Carbohydrates, Increase Water Intake
Leading Causes of Diabetes	
Stress-Emotions (2). Malnutrition (3)	The Brain does not Synchronize Ingested Foods, Medications, Anxiety
Applied Kinesiology	
Helped to a Great Extent (2) Helped to Some Extent (2)	
Number of Clients Who Get Better	
Between 75-85% (2)	About 50%, Between 65-75%,
Indicators of Improvement	
All indicators (4)	

Similarities: Words and Phrases

Type II Diabetes
Obesity (2)
Malnutrition (2)
Dehydration (2)
Stress-Emotions (2)
Pancreatic Damages
Insulin Production (3)
Type I Diabetes
Chromium Assimilation (2)
A damaged chromosome (2)
Gestational Diabetes
Thyroid Weakness (3)
Pre-Diabetic
Obesity (2)
Main Causes of Diabetes
Weight Gain (4)
Dehydration (2)
Environmental Factors
Free radicals (3)
(Ionizing) Radiations (2)
Toxic Particles (2)
Internal Factors or Pathogens
Pathogens (4)
Free Radicals
Obviously, yes (2)
Heavy Metals
Undermine metabolic Procedures (2)
Medications
Liver Dysfunction (2)

Mineral or Vitamin Deficiencies
General Weakness to the Body (2)
A Weak Thyroid
Affect Glandular System (2)
Slows Down Organ Functions (2)
Liver Damaged
Pancreatic damage (3)
Insulin: Resistance
Cell Resistance (2)
Inappropriate Treatment (2)
The Daily Life of Diabetic Patients
No Fruits, Except two of them (2)
Vegetables (2)
No Commercial Juice (2)
Leading Causes of Diabetes
Stress-Emotions (2)
Malnutrition (3)
Applied Kinesiology
Helped to a Great Extent (2)
Helped to some Extent (2)
Number of Clients Who Get Better
Between 75-85% (2)
Indicators of Improvement
All indicators (4)

SUPPLEMENTAL MATERIALS

SUPPLEMENTAL MATERIAL 1

Below is a non-exhaustive list of 17 diabetic super foods, low in carbohydrates and high in fiber.[82]

Food	Serving	Carbs (grams)	Fiber (grams)
1. Avacado	1 medium	17.1	11
2. Artichoke	1 medium	14.3	10.3
3. Lentils	1/2 cup	9.9	7.9
4. Black Beans	1/2 cup	22	7.3
5. Broccoli	1 cup	9	6
6. Oatmeal	1 cup	27	4
7. Barley	1/2 cup	22	3
8. Pumpkin	1 cup, mashed	12	2.9
9. Spinach	1 cup	3.5	2.5
10. Eggplant	1/2 slice	8	2.3
11. Summer Squash	1/2 cup	4	1.9
12. Grapefruit (raw)	1/2 cup sections	10	1.5
13. Tofu, Firm	1/5 pkg.	3	1.5
14. Cauliflower	1/2 cup	2.7	1.3
15. Asparagus	4 spears	2.5	1.2
16. Cabbage	1/2 cup, shredded	3.9	1.2
17. Arugula (raw)	1 cup	2.9	1

Note: The originator of this table measured all the listed foods cooked and unsalted, with the exception of those labeled "raw."

---

[82] The author of the 17 super foods listed above adapted nutritional information based on data from http://www.nutritiondata.com, www.dailyplate.com, www.calorieking.com, and www.mayoclinic.com. Amounts will vary among Brand.

Susan Weiner, R.D., M.S., C.D.E., C.N.D., reviewed the nutritional information, which was last modified on February 7, 2012.

SUPPLEMENTAL MATERIAL 2

16 March 2008

TRUTH ABOUT ASPARTAME

written by: Arthur Evangelista, PhD
former FDA investigator
U.S. Food & Drug Administration—Investigations Branch

BRIEF

While working for the U.S. Food & Drug Administration, I monitored two major projects for FDA, in addition to other product investigations. These projects concerned Pesticides and Chemicals in Foods, and Illegal Drug Tissue Residues in Animals (including milk related issues).

I worked closely with sister federal and state agencies, oversaw contract compliance, and was coordinator and lead investigator on projects involving FDA, EPA, and USDA.

_____

The toxicology, histology, and biochemistry of aspartame (aka: NutraSweet, Equal, etc.) is neurotoxic. The aspartame components injure the blood-brain barrier, allowing easy passage, and will interfere with normal nerve cell function, regardless of whether one is initially symptomatic or not.

Aspartame affects brain tissue, destroying nerve cell integrity, and eventually the neurons, themselves. This leaves lesions or holes where cell death occurred. Aside from brain neurotoxicity, aspartame is known to affect the spinal column nerves, skeletal muscle-nerve junctions, and the conduction system of the heart, as well.

Aspartame is a compound of phenylalanine, aspartic acid, and methanol. The subsequent result from this interaction, and from the isolates of amino acids, is nerve cell necrosis (death), and subsequent organ system disease, along with toxic interactions with many pharmaceutical drugs.

The hypothalamus, the major controller for much of the neuro-endocrine function, is at especially high risk to these effects, and in turn, affects many other organ systems. Thus, the myriad of symptoms.

Methanol (methyl alcohol or wood alcohol) is a colorless, poisonous, and flammable liquid. It is used for making formaldehyde, acetic acid, methyl t-butyl ether (a gasoline additive), and paint strippers. This poison can be inhaled from vapors, absorbed through the skin, and ingested. (Tephly & McMartin 1984)

The methanol in aspartame breaks down into formaldehyde, and formic acid, which denaturizes and mutates the DNA, and can instigate autoimmune disease states. This is a known scientific fact.

PHENYLALANINE (in aspartame) is a free amino acid isolate. Studies show that excessive free phenylalanine damages nerve cells, and is responsible for phenylketonuria in pregnant females. Phenylalanine also reduces serotonin levels in the brain. This reduction in serotonin creates a host of complications. (Wurtman 1988)

Reduced serotonin levels can induce aggressive or violent behavior in adults, and temper tantrums in children. The lowered serotonin level also lowers the threshold for seizure activity, instigating petite and grand mal seizures. (Maher 1987)

The aspartic acid, in aspartame, is a known excitotoxin which easily crosses the blood-brain barrier, and is chemically similar to MSG. An excitotoxin, is a deleterious substance that excites or over stimulates nerve cells to death. (L.E.Rosenberg, McGraw-Hill 1991)

Aspartame creates altered brain function, nerve damage, and systemic organ complications. Information collected by independent research, reveals that aspartame clinically exacerbates any borderline (even yet undetected) predisposing illness, and absolutely complicates certain known medical illnesses like Lupus, Multiple Sclerosis, Parkinson's, diabetes, retinopathies, allergies, and mentation and behavior disorders, et al.

The research data uncovered aspartame's connection regarding nerve cell mitochondria damage, and aspartame-induced brain cell hypoglycemia. Changes in peripheral circulation and nerve transmission occur. Altered systemic metabolites occur, including and the conversion of phenylalanine metabolites into destructive chemical toxins like *diketopiperazine*, a known carcinogen.

Tests reveal a correlation between diketopiperazine and astrocytoma (type of aggressive brain tumor). ASPARTAME is unique in this hazardous respect. Aspartame is not an allergen, but rather, a true toxin.

On the political side and economic perspective, I can only say that politics was the underlying cause of this depraved indifference toward human life, and is exhibited by the FDA-corporate corruption, which had brought aspartame to our tables.

No political or profit based motive should ever replace common sense and the responsibility of preserving the public health . . . EVER. Although, there is no question as to aspartames lethality and instigation of morbidity, ANY question of food safety should ALAWAYS be ruled in favor of public health, until disinterested, third party investigations can be initiated.

From this, it would be apparent, and can be documented, that companies that abstain from using aspartame, have not suffered any financial setbacks.

On the contrary, it would be both re-assuring and publicly acknowledged if a company would actually produce healthy and health supporting foods to the general public.

The publicity of excellent quality controls, acknowledgment of healthful foods, based on scientific and available bio-physiological evidence, would be absolutely welcomed by the consuming public.

This would be especially true, if corporate or federal interference did not place the profit motive before a human being's health needs.

I believe the public requires a governmental body to support the public's best interests and not that of corporate profit motives.

The issues of toxic food additives and their resulting destructive health effects are long term and seriously incapacitating, as earmarked by the number of disease states from the collective insults of foods, air, and water issues, all driven by profit, and distinctly indifferent to common sense health implications.

Make no mistake . . . to rule against aspartame, is to rule in favor of public conviction and good, sound public health principles.

Sincerely,

Arthur M. Evangelista, PhD

Public Health & Medical Fraud
Research Cooperative
P.O. Box 474
Barnardsville, NC 28709
828-658-4174

_____

also see: http://www.thetruthaboutstuff.com/review1.shtml

http://www.thetruthaboutstuff.com/review3.shtml

http://www.aspartame.ca/brain%20cell%20damage.pdf